OTHER *ESSENTIALS* BOOKS

Essentials for the **A&E NURSE**: Guide to a Successful Accident and Emergency Department Orientation, Fourth Edition *(Buettner)*

Essentials on **ADOLESCENT HEALTH FOR NURSING AND HEALTH PROFESSIONALS**: A Care Guide *(Herrman)*

Essentials for the **ADULT-GERONTOLOGY ACUTE CARE NURSE PRACTITIONER** *(Carpenter)*

Essentials for the **ANTEPARTUM AND POSTPARTUM NURSE**: A Nursing Orientation and Care Guide *(Davidson)*

Essentials Workbook for **CARDIAC DYSRHYTHMIAS AND 12-LEAD EKGs** *(Desmarais)*

Essentials for the **CARDIAC SURGERY NURSE**: Caring for Cardiac Surgery Patients, Third Edition *(Hodge)*

Essentials for **CAREER SUCCESS IN NURSING**: Making the Most of Mentoring *(Vance)*

Essentials for the **CATH LAB NURSE** *(McCulloch)*

Essentials for the **CLASSROOM NURSING INSTRUCTOR**: Classroom Teaching *(Yoder-Wise, Kowalski)*

Essentials for the **CLINICAL NURSE LEADER** *(Wilcox, Deerhake)*

Essentials for the **CLINICAL NURSE MANAGER**: Managing a Changing Workplace, Second Edition *(Fry)*

Essentials for the **CLINICAL NURSING INSTRUCTOR**: Clinical Teaching, Third Edition *(Kan, Stabler-Haas)*

Essentials on **COMBATING NURSE BULLYING, INCIVILITY, AND WORKPLACE VIOLENCE**: What Nurses Need to Know *(Ciocco)*

Essentials About **COMPETENCY-BASED EDUCATION IN NURSING**: How to Teach Competency Mastery *(Wittmann-Price, Gittings)*

Essentials for the **CRITICAL CARE NURSE**, Second Edition *(Hewett)*

Essentials About **CURRICULUM DEVELOPMENT IN NURSING**: How to Develop and Evaluate Educational Programs, Second Edition *(McCoy, Anema)*

Essentials for **DEMENTIA CARE**: What Nurses Need to Know, Second Edition *(Miller)*

Essentials for **DEVELOPING A NURSING ACADEMIC PORTFOLIO**: What You Really Need to Know *(Wittmann-Price)*

Essentials for **DNP ROLE DEVELOPMENT**: A Career Navigation Guide *(Menonna-Quinn, Tortorella Genova)*

Essentials About **EKGs FOR NURSES**: The Rules of Identifying EKGs *(Landrum)*

Essentials for **EVIDENCE-BASED PRACTICE IN NURSING**: Third Edition *(Godshall)*

Essentials for the **FAITH COMMUNITY NURSE**: Implementing FCN/Parish Nursing *(Hickman)*

Essentials About **FORENSIC NURSING**: What You Need to Know *(Scannell)*

Essentials for the **GERONTOLOGY NURSE**: A Nursing Care Guide *(Eliopoulos)*

Essentials About **GI AND LIVER DISEASES FOR NURSES**: What APRNs Need to Know *(Chaney)*

Essentials About the **GYNECOLOGICAL EXAM**: A Professional Guide for NPs, PAs, and Midwives, Second Edition *(Secor, Fantasia)*

Essentials in **HEALTH INFORMATICS FOR NURSES** *(Hardy)*

Essentials for **HEALTH PROMOTION IN NURSING**: Promoting Wellness *(Miller)*

Essentials for Nurses About **HOME INFUSION THERAPY**: The Expert's Best Practice Guide *(Gorski)*

Essentials for the **HOSPICE NURSE**: A Concise Guide to End-of-Life Care, Second Edition *(Wright)*

Essentials for the **L&D NURSE**: Labor & Delivery Orientation, Second Edition *(Groll)*

Essentials About **LBGTQ+ CARE FOR NURSES** *(Traister)*

Essentials for the **LONG-TERM CARE NURSE**: What Nursing Home and Assisted Living Nurses Need to Know *(Eliopoulos)*

Essentials to **LOVING YOUR RESEARCH PROJECT**: A Stress-Free Guide for Novice Researchers in Nursing and Healthcare *(Marshall)*

Essentials for **MAKING THE MOST OF YOUR CAREER IN NURSING** *(Redulla)*

Essentials for **MANAGING PATIENTS WITH A PSYCHIATRIC DISORDER**: What RNs, NPs, and New Psych Nurses Need to Know *(Marshall)*

Essentials About **MEDICAL CANNABIS AND OPIOIDS**: Minimizing Opioid Use Through Cannabis *(Smith, Smith)*

Essentials for the **MEDICAL OFFICE NURSE**: What You Really Need to Know *(Richmeier)*

Essentials for the **MEDICAL–SURGICAL NURSE**: Clinical Orientation *(Ciocco)*

Essentials for the **NEONATAL NURSE**: Care Essentials for Normal and High-Risk Neonates, Second Edition *(Davidson)*

Essentials About **NEUROCRITICAL CARE**: A Quick Reference for the Advanced Practice Provider *(McLaughlin)*

Essentials for the **NEW NURSE PRACTITIONER**: What You Really Need to Know, Second Edition *(Aktan)*

Essentials for **NURSE PRACTITIONERS:** Practice Essentials for Clinical Subspecialties *(Aktan)*

Essentials for the **NURSE PRECEPTOR**: Keys to Providing a Successful Preceptorship, Second Edition *(Ciocco)*

Essentials for the **NURSE PSYCHOTHERAPIST**: The Process of Becoming *(Jones, Tusaie)*

Essentials About **NURSING AND THE LAW**: Law for Nurses *(Grant, Ballard)*

Essentials About the **NURSING PROFESSION**: Historical Perspectives *(Hunt)*

Essentials for the **OPERATING ROOM NURSE**: An Orientation and Care Guide, Second Edition *(Criscitelli)*

Essentials for the **PEDIATRIC NURSE**: An Orientation Guide *(Rupert, Young)*

Essentials Handbook for **PEDIATRIC PRIMARY CARE:** A Guide for Nurse Practitioners and Physician Assistants *(Ruggiero, Ruggiero)*

Essentials About **PRESSURE ULCER CARE FOR NURSES**: How to Prevent, Detect, and Resolve Them *(Dziedzic)*

Essentials About **PTSD**: A Guide for Nurses and Other Health Care Professionals *(Adams)*

Essentials for the **RADIOLOGY NURSE**: An Orientation and Nursing Care Guide, Second Edition *(Grossman)*

Essentials About **RELIGION FOR NURSES**: Implications for Patient Care *(Taylor)*

Essentials for the **SCHOOL NURSE**: What You Need to Know, Third Edition *(Loschiavo)*

Essentials About **SEXUALLY TRANSMITTED INFECTIONS**: A Nurse's Guide to Expert Patient Care *(Scannell)*

Essentials for **STROKE CARE NURSING**: An Expert Care Guide, Second Edition *(Morrison)*

Essentials for the **STUDENT NURSE**: Nursing Student Success *(Stabler-Haas)*

Essentials About **SUBSTANCE USE DISORDERS**: What Every Nurse, APRN, and PA Needs to Know *(Marshall, Spencer)*

Essentials for the **TRAVEL NURSE**: Travel Nursing *(Landrum)*

Essentials for the **TRIAGE NURSE**: An Orientation and Care Guide, Second Edition *(Visser, Montejano)*

Essentials for **WOUND CARE NURSING** *(Myers)*

Essentials for **WRITING THE DNP PROJECT**: Effective Structure, Content, and Presentation *(Christenbery)*

ESSENTIALS for
THE OR NURSE

Theresa Criscitelli, EdD, RN, CNOR, is a doctorally prepared nurse who has spent 26 years working in the operating room. Her career began as a certified surgical technologist when she learned to scrub in on an array of surgical specialties, including neurosurgery, orthopedics, and cardiothoracic open-heart surgery. She completed her nursing degree in order to care for surgical patients as their advocate and to be able to obtain other positions in the perioperative area that could help influence patient outcomes. She has held numerous positions in the perioperative setting as a registered nurse, including staff nurse, assistant nurse manager, nurse educator, director of perioperative education, and assistant director of professional nursing practice and education. Dr. Criscitelli is currently working in administration and oversees the perioperative and procedural services at a major hospital in New York. She also serves as adjunct nursing professor at three colleges and was a clinical instructor in a surgical technology program. She has participated with research and continues to mentor students and staff.

Her love for the perioperative field does not cease at the end of the workday. She has published numerous articles in journals and has conducted research on the operating room that has been presented internationally. She oversees an operating room fellowship program and helped establish an academic-service partnership at a local university to provide a capstone experience in the operating room for undergraduate nursing students during their senior year. Engaging new nurses in the perioperative setting is her aspiration.

ESSENTIALS for **THE OR NURSE**

An Orientation and Care Guide

Third Edition

Theresa Criscitelli, EdD, RN, CNOR

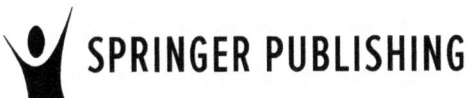

Copyright © 2022 Springer Publishing Company, LLC

All rights reserved.
First Springer publishing edition 2015; subsequent edition 2018

No part of this publication may be reproduced, stored in a retrieval system, or transmitted in any form or by any means, electronic, mechanical, photocopying, recording, or otherwise, without the prior permission of Springer Publishing Company, LLC, or authorization through payment of the appropriate fees to the Copyright Clearance Center, Inc., 222 Rosewood Drive, Danvers, MA 01923, 978-750-8400, fax 978-646-8600, info@copyright.com or on the Web at www.copyright.com.

Springer Publishing Company, LLC
11 West 42nd Street
New York, NY 10036
www.springerpub.com

Acquisitions Editor: Rachel X. Landes
Compositor: Transforma

ISBN: 978-0-8261-6712-5

The author and the publisher of this Work have made every effort to use sources believed to be reliable to provide information that is accurate and compatible with the standards generally accepted at the time of publication. Because medical science is continually advancing, our knowledge base continues to expand. Therefore, as new information becomes available, changes in procedures become necessary. We recommend that the reader always consult current research and specific institutional policies before performing any clinical procedure. The author and publisher shall not be liable for any special, consequential, or exemplary damages resulting, in whole or in part, from the readers' use of, or reliance on, the information contained in this book. The publisher has no responsibility for the persistence or accuracy of URLs for external or third-party Internet websites referred to in this publication and does not guarantee that any content on such websites is, or will remain, accurate or appropriate.

The *Essentials* series was published in the United States of America as the *Fast Facts* series.

Contents

Foreword Kay Ball, PhD, RN, CNOR, CMSLO, FAAN ix
Preface xi
Acknowledgments xiii
Introduction xv

PERSONAL AND PATIENT PREPARATION

1. Surgical Attire 3
2. Preoperative Considerations 13
3. Patient Positioning 23
4. Surgical Skin Preparation 35
5. Draping the Patient for Surgery 41

ENVIRONMENT AND PROCESSING CONSIDERATIONS

6. Operating Room Environment Requirements 51
7. Sterile Technique 59
8. Sterilization and Central Processing 71
9. Surgical Supplies 83

Part III SURGICAL BASICS

10. Basic Surgical Procedures	95
11. Surgical Instrumentation	109
12. Electrosurgery	121
13. Surgical Energy and Stapling Devices	131
14. Surgical Dressings	139

Part IV ADDITIONAL OPERATING ROOM CONSIDERATIONS

15. Medications	149
16. Anesthesia	155
17. Complications and Emergencies in the Operating Room	165
18. Emergency Preparedness for Disaster	177
19. Legal Aspects of Operating Room Practice	185
20. Lifelong Learning	191

Bibliography	*199*
Index	*203*

Foreword

Every decade the perioperative environment changes significantly, mandating that surgical team members remain current with their skills and knowledge. Patient safety continues to be the foundation upon which this ever-changing arena is based. Evidence-based practices evolve from this foundation as new research lights the path to excellence in perioperative practice. A comprehensive orientation to surgical settings and patient care is mandatory in this fast-paced environment so that learning is unique, all-inclusive, and logical. Therefore, vital to any perioperative educational program is a comprehensive reference book with content that enhances the skill level and knowledge of all surgical team members.

Essentials for the OR Nurse: An Orientation and Care Guide by Theresa Criscitelli, EdD, RN, CNOR, is a very handy reference book with vital information that is easy to access, understand, and implement. Perioperative nurses and surgical technologists, whether they are being oriented to the operating room or are skilled healthcare providers, can use this book to guide their surgical practices. Students in academia who are being introduced to perioperative practices will find this book to be a valuable resource in their educational processes.

The format for this reference book is based on the three critical themes of "Personal and Patient Preparation," "Environment and Processing Considerations," and "Surgical Basics." While focusing on patient safety and recommended perioperative practices, the all-inclusive skills required in circulating and scrubbing are highlighted. Explanations and details about surgical techniques, practices, and patient care are provided in concise, step-by-step, logical formats, with illustrations and diagrams to enhance learning. Evidence-based content that is built on current standards, guidelines, and recommended practices is highlighted to promote patient safety and excellence in the perioperative setting.

This easy-to-use reference book is a vital resource for every surgical suite and academic perioperative program. The book fits nicely into a pocket for easy retrieval and reference during the challenging days in the OR. Any perioperative professional will find this enhanced edition provides the valuable education and information required for critical thinking and clinical reasoning in the perioperative environment. This book is a must for updated learning and comprehensive orientation to the perioperative setting!

Kay Ball, PhD, RN, CNOR, CMSLO, FAAN
Professor, Nursing
Otterbein University, Westerville, Ohio
Past President, Association of periOperative Registered Nurses

Preface

Essentials for the OR Nurse can be the perfect companion for the registered nurse (RN), certified surgical technologist (CST), or RN first assistant. The *Essentials* series provides essential nursing facts that are needed daily to provide the best practices to each and every patient. This book condenses volumes of operating room content into one handy book that can be tucked away and concealed in a scrub-jacket pocket.

The new RN who comes to the operating room for an orientation program can use this book to better understand complex skills and techniques, which are presented in a very simple and easy-to-follow format. The experienced perioperative nurse can also benefit from this book. Many practices have changed over the years, making it difficult to keep up with the current standards. The third edition of *Essentials for the OR Nurse* provides the up-to-date information necessary to practice in this evidence-based environment. Why cull over multiple textbooks, articles, and guidelines to find the information that you need? Let this *Essentials* series volume be your resource. Although this book is not a comprehensive resource, if more in-depth information is needed for any of the book's topics, other sources can be consulted. There are many other excellent resources available to provide additional details.

Preceptors can recommend this book to their learners to provide an evidence-based approach to assist in ensuring competent nursing practice. It can also be utilized by new graduates, new hires, or even the onboarding of nurses to the operating room, which may be a new clinical setting for them. This book can provide the perfect content to reinforce safety and current knowledge relative to perioperative standards.

This book is divided into four sections, beginning with information on preparing yourself and your patient for surgery. Then it extends into all of the relevant facts related to the practice environment of the operating room and the processing of equipment and supplies. The next few chapters discuss surgical procedures and instrumentation. There is a great deal to understand about actual surgical procedures and the devices used during them. Finally, the section on additional operating room considerations provides further information on other important aspects of operating room nursing and includes two new chapters on Emergency Preparedness for Disaster and Lifelong Learning.

Each chapter introduces concepts and sets clear, obtainable learning objectives. The Essentials boxes provide self-assessment questions to help test your knowledge as you go along to see how much you are really learning. These boxes also provide pearls of wisdom—critical pieces of information highlighted for easy access. The tables allow quick reference, so you can find common information quickly and easily when needed. The language of this book is simple and clear, so that complex facts can be easily understood by not only the seasoned nurse, but also the new operating room nurse.

Theresa Criscitelli

Acknowledgments

I would like to thank all of the operating room friends and students I have met along my journey. Special thanks to Dr. Gary Sher, who has always been there through many of my life events to encourage me and assist in guiding my viewpoint on life. I would also like to thank Andrea Jahn, CRCST, and Kristine Nawrocki, CRCST, for not only being a great colleagues and friends, but also for their vast knowledge and love of central sterile. This book would not have been possible without the love and support from my husband, Perry, who encourages me every step of the way, and is my best friend. Most importantly, I wish to thank my two wonderful children, Walter and Benjamin, who provide never-ending inspiration.

Introduction

The operating room is a fast-paced, technological environment wherein the perioperative registered nurse (RN) must be able to think quickly and accurately, as well as advocate for the patient while the patient is under anesthesia. Working in the operating room is a privilege, and it should always be looked upon as an honor to be the nurse providing optimal care to the surgical patient. This requires the nurse to use not only his or her basic nursing skills, but to have the additional skills of aseptic technique, knowledge of surgical procedures, and familiarity with the specialized equipment—all skills that are many times learned on the job.

The orientation to the operating room can be an overwhelming experience, filled with anxiety, unexpected events, and sometimes even tears; however, those experiences can be mitigated through preparation. Therefore, a comprehensive orientation is necessary to nurture and guide the new operating room nurse in this exciting environment. So, if you do not know where operating room nurses come from, how would you know where they are going? Therefore, understanding the history of the operating room nurse can help define where these nurses are today and where they are going in the future.

In the early 18th century, operating rooms were basically large, crowded areas containing sick patients and a great deal of cluttered medical supplies. This resulted in high infection rates, so a drastic change took place late in the 18th century, when operating rooms became separate spaces and the operating theater was introduced. This amphitheater allowed people to watch the surgeries as they took place, and, in the 1870s and 1880s, became a form of entertainment for the wealthy.

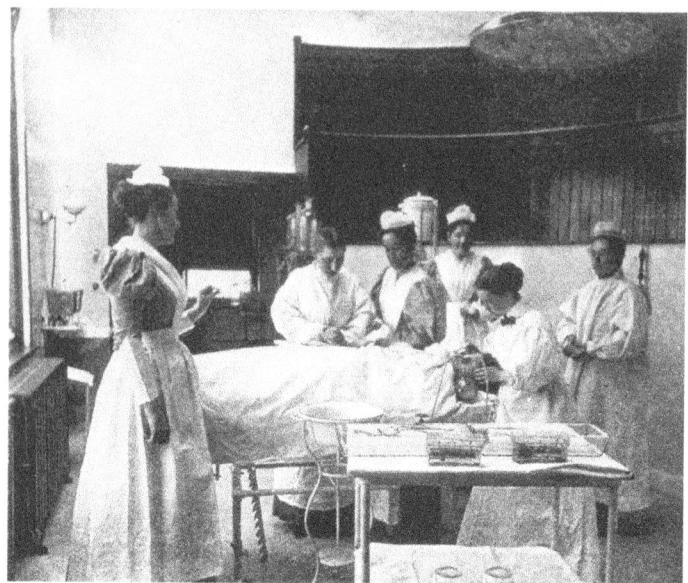

Operating Theatre: Brooklyn Memorial Hospital for Women and Children (1898).
Source: U.S. National Library of Medicine. New York, NY: W. Abbatt.

In the 1890s, the position of surgical nurse evolved, which is now known as the "operating room nurse." The surgical nurse was given specific lectures on preparing a patient for surgery, assisting the surgeon during surgery, surgical emergencies, and the preparation of dressings. Surgeons realized the value that a nurse could provide in the operating room setting. Someone who knew the procedures, the instruments, and the necessary dressings was a welcome addition to this environment.

As time went on, in the early part of the 20th century, little was known about bacteria and germs, and, in an effort to reduce infection, nurses spent many hours cleaning and sterilizing instruments and surgical items for reuse. The Spanish-flu pandemic of 1918 brought about the use of cotton masks in the operating room. Until then, doctors and nurses wore only aprons to protect their clothing or uniforms from being soiled. Gowns and gloves were cleaned and then sterilized after each use.

Operating room attire was originally white to represent cleanliness, but changed to green by the 1960s when it was discovered that the white scrubs caused eyestrain for the surgeons. Also, instruments were washed in soap and water, and then placed in carbolic acid to soak. This sterilized the instruments and it was found to reduce postoperative infections. Before 1960, sutures were made from sheep or cattle intestines and were called "gut" sutures. These were the most popular type and were hand threaded onto a free suture needle.

Times have changed, and now the operating room is a highly restricted area with numerous regulatory guidelines, specialized technology, and myriad opportunities for both the new operating room nurse and the seasoned professional. Working in the operating room is an interprofessional collaboration involving many roles. Within the scope of the RN, the nurse can take part either as the scrub or as the circulating nurse.

The scrub nurse is responsible for:

- Preparing the room for surgery, including maintaining the sterile field
- Passing instruments to the surgical team
- Preparing medications and other items on the sterile field
- Assisting in the safe transfer of the surgical patient to the postanesthesia care unit

The scrub nurse is gowned and gloved during the procedure and many times assists the surgeon. The certified surgical technologist (CST) can also perform the role of the scrub nurse and, in some states, can perform some circulating nursing roles. It is important to know the policy of the institution regarding each role's job description.

The circulating nurse is responsible for:

- Preparing the patient and the room for surgery
- Assisting in the positioning of the patient
- Assisting the anesthesia care provider
- Completing the nursing documentation
- Acquiring any additional items that need to be provided for surgery

The circulating nurse may leave the operating room for short periods of time to get things that are needed, but along with the surgical team, the nurse is responsible for the patient.

Other members of the surgical team include but are not limited to:

- Attending surgeon
- Additional surgeons
- Anesthesiologist
- Nurse anesthetist
- RN first assistant
- CST
- Residents
- Medical school students
- Physician assistants
- Nurse practitioners
- Unit support personnel

It is important to know exactly who is in the operating room and to try to keep the amount of personnel as low as possible. The surgical suite can become very crowded at times.

It is essential to realize that surgery does not always take place in the hospital. Over the past decade, more and more surgical procedures are being performed in ambulatory care units and centers. Also, doctors have opened up operating rooms in their offices, which must also adhere to strict sterile techniques to prevent surgical-site infections. Many of the basic concepts within this book apply to the very different environments in which an operating room can now be found.

The Association of periOperative Registered Nurses (AORN) is the national organization for operating room nurses. It is important to be part of the national organization in order to:

- Stay current on specific issues
- Effect legislation within your state
- Stay connected to a network of nurses across the country
- Engage in educational opportunities

It is not only important to be part of an organization, but furthering your knowledge within your specialty is equally as important. A specialty nursing certification can be obtained called "CNOR." This is the gold standard of operating room nursing. CNOR is not an acronym but is considered "the documented validation of the professional achievement of identified standards of practice by an individual RN providing care for patients before, during and after surgery" (Competency & Credentialing Institute, n.d.). CNOR certification can be obtained by sitting for an examination after completing a minimum of 2 years or 2,400 hours of experience in perioperative nursing, with a minimum of 50% (1,200 hours) spent in the intraoperative setting.

The pathway to certification and the importance of membership in a nationally recognized organization, such as AORN, are exciting, and support the RNs' practice in the operating room. The benefits of belonging to AORN range from the opportunity for grants and scholarships, to connecting with other operating room nurses around the world. As you embark upon your journey as an operating room nurse, remember to stay engaged in not only what is going on at your personal institution, but what is going on around the nation and the world.

Reference

Competency & Credentialing Institute. (n.d.). About CNOR. Retrieved from http://www.cc-institute.org/cnor/about

I

Personal and Patient Preparation

1

Surgical Attire

Surgical attire is the first aspect of preparation for a day in the operating room. It is important to adhere to specific surgical attire standards that will promote a safe environment and ensure cleanliness. Personnel should change into surgical attire in a dressing room that is close to the semi-restricted and restricted areas of the operating room. This will prevent contamination of attire and limit the amount of traffic with those in street clothing or anyone from the external environment.

During this part of your orientation, you will learn about:

- The acceptable attire to wear and why
- What not to wear and why
- Related concerns regarding safety and transmission of microorganisms

CONTROLLED AREAS

The surgical environment is a controlled-traffic area that is monitored regarding patients, family, personnel, and materials. Signage should clearly define the surgical attire required.

Restricted area: This is an area restricted to specific personnel and patients because a sterile field is established in this area and must be monitored. Also, this area contains specialized equipment that is delicate and expensive. Scrubs must be worn, hair covered, and masks worn, if a sterile field is opened. Examples of restricted areas include operating room suites and scrub sink areas.

Semirestricted area: This is an area that is restricted to specific personnel and patients, but not where sterile fields are established. Scrubs must be worn and hair covered. Examples of semirestricted areas include storage areas, areas for the processing of instruments, and utility areas.

Transition area: This is an area adjacent to the semirestricted or restricted area where staff can enter in street clothing and then exit in scrubs. An example of a transition area is the locker room.

Monitored unrestricted area: This is an area where patients, families, and staff are permitted. The staff would be in scrubs, the patient in a gown, and the family in street clothing. Examples of monitored unrestricted areas include the preoperative holding area and the postanesthesia care unit.

SCRUBS

Description of Scrubs

- Scrubs consist of a scrub top and scrub pants.
- The top should be tucked into the pants to prevent skin cells from shedding.
- The drawstring waist should be tied and tucked in to prevent the strings from flapping around and contaminating the sterile field.
- Scrubs should be made of a low-lint and tightly woven material.
- Scrubs should be made of durable and stain-resistant material that has a low flammability rate.
- Fleece material is not recommended. Fleece may be warm, but it is highly flammable, can shed lint, accumulates dust and skin, and harbors moisture.
- Disposable scrubs are another alternative and must be discarded at the end of the day.
- Scrubs should not fit too loosely or too tightly. This will ensure a professional look.

The Do Nots of Scrubs

- Scrubs should not be in a locker where they may be exposed to personal clothing, pocketbooks, food, or any outside items.
- No undergarments should extend out of the neckline or sleeve line of the scrub top.
- Soiled or wet scrubs should not be worn. They should be changed as soon as possible to prevent exposure to pathogens.

Laundering of Scrubs

- Laundering should occur at a healthcare-accredited laundry facility (Table 1.1).
- It is important to know the type of washer, the water temperature, the laundry soap strength, and the rinse cycle; this will ensure that the scrubs that are placed against the perioperative personnel's skin are clean and free of microorganisms.
- Due to the increasing number of resistant bacteria and their ability to survive, the home laundry cycle can transfer bacteria or pathogens to other fabrics and subsequent loads.

Essential Facts

Home laundering of scrubs is not recommended. Remember, the operating room is a source of microbial transmission and contamination.

Table 1.1

Healthcare-Accredited Laundering Requirements

Cycle	Temperature	Time	Action
Wash	At least 160°F (71°C)	At least 25 min	Mechanical, thermal, chemical
Chlorine bleach or oxygen-based bleach	135°F–145°F (57.2°C–62.7°C)	Until chlorine residual of 50–150 parts per million (ppm) achieved	Mechanical, thermal, chemical
Rinse	pH 5–12	Dictated by manufacturer	Neutralizes alkalinity
Dry	At least 180°F (82°C)	Dictated by fabric	Thermal
Press/iron	State regulated	Dictated by fabric	Thermal

> **Essential Facts**
>
> **Question:** Why should surgical attire be laundered by an accredited laundry facility?
> **Answer:** *It establishes quality controls and monitoring and prevents contamination of personnel's own washers and dryers.*

HEAD COVERINGS

Head coverings, such as a bouffant hat (Figure 1.1), should cover the perioperative personnel's hair. If there is facial hair, sideburns, or neck hair, it must also be covered. This will prevent the shedding of hair and skin cells from the scalp and other areas that can potentially contaminate the surgical environment. Head covers must be changed daily, and if the head cover is made of scrub material, it must be laundered daily at a healthcare-accredited laundry facility.

The Do Nots of Head Coverings

- Skull caps (Figure 1.2) are not recommended because they do not cover well.
- Never wear a head covering that allows hair to protrude.
- Never rewear cloth hats without proper washing at a healthcare-accredited laundry facility.

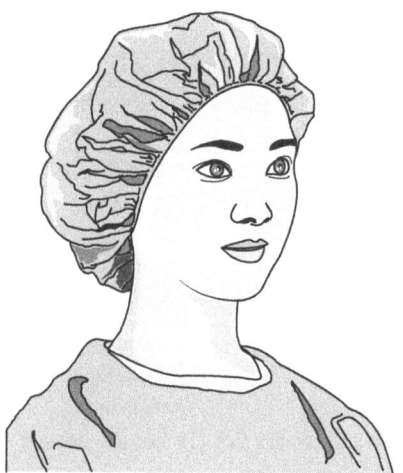

Figure 1.1 Bouffant style.

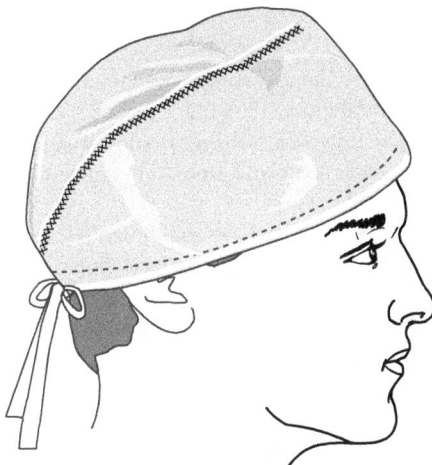

Figure 1.2 Skull-cap style.

SCRUB JACKETS

Scrub jackets should be made of the same material as scrubs and be limited to 1 day of use. The scrub jacket should have long sleeves and snaps. Non-scrubbed personnel are encouraged to wear a scrub jacket, not only because the operating room may be cool, but to prevent skin shedding from the arms. This will also protect the non-scrubbed personnel from liquids or body fluids splashing onto their bare arms. Another option is a disposable scrub jacket that can be thrown away at the end of the day.

The Do Nots of Scrub Jackets

- Do not wear fleece scrub jacket materials.
- Do not home launder scrub jackets.
- Do not leave the scrub jacket unsnapped whereby the edge of the jacket can flap and contaminate the sterile field.

Essential Facts

Question: How should scrub jackets be worn?
Answer: Scrub jackets should be snapped closed, cuffed at the wrists, and only worn for 1 day.

SHOES

Shoes that are worn in the operating room should be worn only in that setting. No one should wear the same shoes outside and/or at home. Wearing those shoes in other settings would spread microorganisms and debris to outside areas and would also introduce microorganisms and debris from outside.

Shoes should have a closed toe and closed back, a low heel, and soles made of a nonskid material to prevent slipping or tripping. The top surface of the shoe should not have any holes or perforations, to prevent blood and body fluids, liquids, or sharp objects from penetrating the perioperative personnel's skin.

The Do Nots of Shoes

- Cloth shoes should not be worn in the operating room because they are porous and cannot be easily cleaned.
- Clogs without a secure back should not be worn, due to the potential for tripping.
- Crocs™, although fashionable, should not be worn, due to the lack of support and the fenestrations on the top surface.

SHOE COVERS

Shoe covers come in different lengths, beginning with covers that just cover the shoe. They may also be longer and cover up to the knee. They are made of an impervious material to prevent fluid penetration and absorption. Shoe covers are recommended when the surgical procedure may result in extensive fluid release. Shoe covers should be worn over any shoes that are worn outside of the hospital or healthcare facility.

The Do Nots of Shoe Covers

- Shoe covers should not be worn outside of the transition area into the overall hospital setting.
- Shoe covers should not be worn when visibly soiled or saturated with fluids.
- Shoe covers should not be taken off with bare hands; utility gloves must be worn when discarding shoe covers.

ADDITIONAL ITEMS

Jewelry

Jewelry, including but not limited to earrings, necklaces, watches, bracelets, and body piercings, should not be worn in the operating room due to the high risk of contamination. The cracks and crevices in jewelry harbor bacteria that can spread in the healthcare setting and in patients. Another safety concern is the chance of injury as jewelry may become caught on equipment, fabric, or patients.

Essential Facts

Research has shown that bacterial counts are nine times higher on the skin beneath rings than on skin that does not have any jewelry on it.

Stethoscopes

Stethoscopes, although essential for some operating room personnel, should not be worn around the neck. They must be cleaned between patients. They are an inanimate object that can transmit pathogens by indirect contact.

Identification Badges

The identification badge should be worn to identify all personnel and to determine whether they are authorized to be in the surgical area or even the hospital. This practice will help maintain a safe environment and deter unauthorized visitors. Vendors and visitors may be provided with a 1-day pass or be required to use an automated badge terminal. This terminal will check the vendor's credentials and health records before printing out an identification pass.

One-day identification badges should contain:

- Date
- Time
- Photo
- Company information
- Name
- Areas of access

Personal Items

Any personal items that are brought into the operating room must be cleaned with a low-level disinfectant and should not be placed on the floor. If the item is difficult or impossible to clean, and the item is necessary in the operating room, it must be placed in a clean plastic bag while in the operating room.

Personal items include:

- Briefcase
- Backpack
- Cellphone
- Tablet

Masks

The surgical mask protects the patient and the perioperative personnel from being exposed to germs. Wearing a mask prevents droplets greater than 5 microns from being inhaled or exhaled. A surgical N95 respirator or higher-level respirator may be required depending upon the patient condition and procedure performed.

- Masks should cover the nose and mouth.
- Masks are secured behind the head and at the neck.
- A mask should be tight enough to prevent space at the sides.
- A mask should not be worn around the neck or have the strings hanging.
- Masks should be changed when they are soiled or wet.
- After changing a mask, hands should be washed with soap and water to prevent contamination.

Because eye protection is recommended, a mask with an attached fluid shield (Figure 1.3) is one option that can be disposed of after each surgery. It also provides protection around the sides of the face.

Essential Facts

It is difficult for beginners to get used to wearing a surgical mask. You may feel as though you cannot breathe or that you are going to pass out. Stay calm. You will get acclimated to its use in a few weeks.

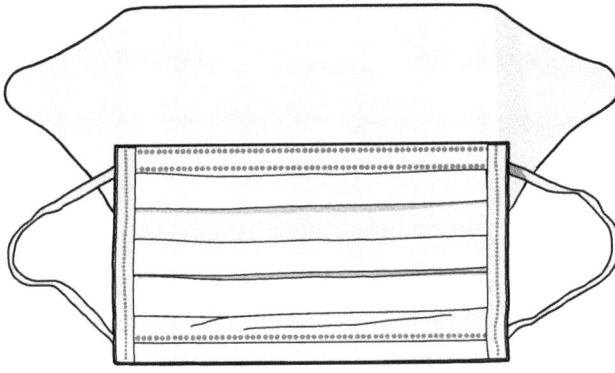

Figure 1.3 Mask with fluid shield.

INFECTION CONTROL CONCERNS

Surgical personnel who must leave the operating room area may be asked to wear a cover coat. This protocol should be regulated by the institution's infection control department. Doctors and nurses who go to patient rooms, the cafeteria, or another department within the hospital may have to don a cover coat.

If surgical personnel need to travel to another healthcare facility, they must change from surgical attire into street clothing and don clean surgical attire at the next facility. This will prevent the transfer of pathogens.

2

Preoperative Considerations

The preoperative period for a patient is an important time to ensure that the patient is physically and psychologically ready for surgery. Patients who are prepared tend to have a better hospital experience and a more positive surgical outcome. If the surgical procedure is planned and not emergent, this can be a time for education, information gathering, and careful planning.

During this part of your orientation, you will learn about:

- The preoperative considerations for surgical patients
- How to conduct a preoperative assessment
- Important regulatory requirements
- Preoperative warming of the surgical patient

THE FIRST STEP: THE PREOPERATIVE SHOWER

The Centers for Medicare & Medicaid Services have adopted payment rules that went into effect in 2008 that deny reimbursement for surgical-site infections (SSIs). Therefore, surgical patients should be instructed to perform a preoperative shower or bath the night before surgery and the morning of surgery. This involves the use of 2% or 4% chlorhexidine gluconate (CHG) soap to decrease the amount of microorganisms on the patient's body, ultimately reducing the bacterial count and the chance of acquiring an SSI. For convenience and patients who cannot get out of bed, 2% CHG no-rinse disposable cloths can be used. These cloths should be used by wiping skin surfaces and allowing the product to dry on the skin.

Patient Procedure

- Wash with soap and water.
- Wash with 2% or 4% CHG soap.
- Do not use the CHG soap above the neck, on the genitals, or on any mucous membrane.
- Dry with a clean towel.
- Apply clean clothing and use clean sheets.
- Do not apply any lotions, deodorants, powders, perfumes, or colognes after washing.
- Do not apply any alcohol-based hair or skin products that can cause a fire hazard in the operating room.

PREOPERATIVE MEDICATIONS

Depending upon the type of surgery and the patient's history, the physician or anesthesia provider may order medications. These are commonly antibiotics, to prevent SSI, or sedatives, to relax the patient prior to surgery. Other medications may be ordered dependent upon specific patient situations.

Antibiotics

Antibiotics should be given prophylactically within 1 hour before surgical incision. The type of antibiotic is most often based upon the type of procedure the patient is having. This is called *procedure-based antibiotics* and they are stopped 24 hours after the anesthesia has ended, unless the surgeon provides a rationale to continue.

Common preoperative antibiotics are:

- Cefazolin
- Levofloxacin
- Vancomycin (will be given over a longer period of time)

Sedatives

Sedation may be ordered before surgery to relax the patient. If sedation is ordered, depending upon the medication, additional monitoring may be required. Also, the patient may not be able to walk into the operating room if in an ambulatory setting.

Common sedation medications are:

- Diazepam
- Midazolam
- Hydroxyzine

IDENTIFICATION OF THE PATIENT

The surgical patient must be identified whenever approached, even if you know who the patient is. It is imperative to use two identifiers, which will be determined by your healthcare facility.

Examples of patient identifiers are:

- Name
- Date of birth
- Medical record number

PREOPERATIVE QUESTIONS

It is important to complete a thorough preoperative nursing assessment. The questioning of the surgical patient should be done in a nonthreatening, calm, and concise way. Time must be taken to probe into any inconsistencies or concerns. Components of the nursing assessment and documentation may vary dependent upon the healthcare facility.

Common components are:

- Nothing-by-mouth (NPO) status
- Allergies
- Physical examination
- Past medical history
- Past surgical history
- Past psychosocial history
- Medications/herbal supplements[1] currently taking
- Fractures and skeletal limitations
- Contact lenses, jewelry, body piercings, prosthetics, dentures
- Pain assessment

---

[1] Herbal supplements are just as potent as medications and many times not mentioned during a patient assessment.

Essential Facts

Question: What should you do if the patient tells you that he ate a light meal the morning of surgery?
Answer: Ask the patient what time he ate and tell the anesthesia care provider and the surgeon. This may delay the surgery.

Herbal supplements can:

- Increase bleeding
- Interact with other medications
- Have an increased sedating effect
- Be associated with cardiovascular risks

Some herbal supplements that increase bleeding are:

- Gingko biloba
- Garlic
- Ginseng
- Fish oil
- Dong quai
- Feverfew

PREOPERATIVE TEACHING

Preoperative teaching must be individualized dependent upon many factors, such as:

- Age
- Educational level
- Cultural beliefs
- Religious beliefs
- Mental status

It is important to address the patient's plan of care and also address questions from the family.

Components of teaching:

- Describe what will happen and how the patient may feel postoperatively.
- Discuss the length of the procedure and postoperative recovery time.
- Alleviate fears or anxiety.
- Explain expectations of postoperative pain and medications available.
- Answer any questions.

Essential Facts

If the patient expresses fear of dying related to the surgical procedure, it is recommended to share this information with the attending physician prior to bringing the patient into the operating room. Then the physician can discuss this with the patient prior to going forward with the procedure.

LAB WORK

Lab work will vary within different institutions and is dependent upon several factors, such as:

- Patient age
- Patient gender
- Surgical procedure
- Physician
- Health history
- Surgical history
- Treatment history

Table 2.1 lists common lab tests for adults.

Table 2.1

Common Lab Tests for Adults

Name of Lab Test	Abbreviation	Common Acceptable Range
Red blood cells	RBC	4.2–5.5 mcL
White blood cells	WBC	4–11 mcL
Hemoglobin	HGB	12–18 gm/dL
Hematocrit	HCT	37%–47%
Platelets	PLT	140–440 mcL
Prothrombin time	PT	11–14 sec
Partial thromboplastin time	PTT	18–41 sec
International normalized ratio	INR	0.8–1.2
Platelets	PLT	140–440
Potassium	K	3.5–5 mEq/L
Sodium	Na	135–145 mEq/L

(continued)

Table 2.1

Common Lab Tests for Adults (continued)

Name of Lab Test	Abbreviation	Common Acceptable Range
Chloride	Cl	100–106 mEq/L
Glucose	GLU	70–110 mg/mL
Creatinine	CR	0.2–0.9 mg/dL
Carbon dioxide	CO_2	24–30 mEq/L
Blood urea nitrogen	BUN	8–25 mg/100 mL
Digoxin	DIG	0.8–2 ng/mL

The ranges of each lab test can vary depending upon age, gender, and healthcare facility recommendations.

INFORMED CONSENT

By law, the physician who is performing the surgical procedure must obtain informed consent from the patient. This means that the patient must understand the risks, benefits, and alternatives to the surgery. The patient should be given time to ask questions and determine what is the best choice.

To sign a consent form, the patient must be:

- 18 years old or older
- Not mentally impaired, due to disability or medication
- If not 18 years or older, an emancipated minor, who is a person under 18 years of age who has been granted independence from his or her parent(s) by a court of law (each state has specific emancipation statutes or procedural rules)

If the patient cannot sign the consent form, the persons eligible to sign are:

- Next of kin, being a spouse, adult child, or adult sibling
- Person with power of attorney or healthcare proxy
- For children under 18 years of age, a parent or legal guardian

Essential Facts

Power of attorney is the legal permission for another person to make decisions on the patient's behalf. A healthcare proxy grants

(continued)

(*continued*)

permission to a designated person to act on the patient's behalf in the event of incapacitation.

UNIVERSAL PROTOCOL

The Joint Commission Board of Commissioners requires all accredited hospitals, ambulatory care, and office-based surgical facilities to utilize universal protocol (UP) to prevent wrong-site, wrong-procedure, and wrong-person surgery.

There are three elements to UP:

1. Preprocedural Verification
   This is to ensure that all of the important documents and studies are available and have been reviewed before the surgery starts. Any missing or discrepant information must be addressed at this point. Everyone on the surgical team must agree that:
   - The patient whom they are operating on is correct
   - The procedure that they are performing is correct
   - The accurate site of surgery is correct
   - The studies are correct for the patient and procedure
   - The implants, if any, are available in the operating room and are correct
   - The plan of care, which includes anesthetic plan, blood loss, and anything unique to the patient, is appropriate

2. Site Marking
   This is to clearly indicate the intended site of the incision or insertion. This includes the physician's indelible marking, which is to be clearly visible after the patient is draped and must be done when procedures involve:
   - Right or left distinction
   - Multiple structures, such as toes or fingers
   - Multiple levels in spine surgery

3. Time Out (takes place in the operating room)
   This is a final verification that *all* members of the surgical team must pause and participate in, and includes verification of:
   - The correct patient, procedure, and site marked and visible
   - Fire risk discussed
   - Relevant images properly labeled and displayed
   - Any equipment concerns
   - Any anticipated critical events

- Prophylactic antibiotics given
- Sterilization indicators checked and confirmed

4. Sign Out
   - This is performed before the surgeon and the patient leaves the operating room and includes verification of:
   - Name of operative procedure
   - Completion of counts
   - Specimen identification and labeling confirmation
   - Discussion of wound classification
   - Equipment problems addressed
   - Recovery management concerns

PREOPERATIVE WARMING

It is important to prevent inadvertent perioperative hypothermia. *Hypothermia* occurs when the core body temperature is below 96.8°F (36°C). Therefore, it is desirable to keep the patient normothermic. *Normothermic* refers to as core body temperature between 96.8°F and 100.4°F (36°C and 38°C) (Giuliano & Hendricks, 2017).

Prewarming of patients for at least 15 minutes prior to surgery can prevent the loss of body heat that is common during surgical procedures. Patients who should be prewarmed include:

- Neonates and infants
- The elderly
- Patients with low body weight
- Patients with metabolic disorders
- Patients taking antipsychotics or antidepressants
- Patients undergoing procedures using a pneumatic tourniquet
- Patients having open-cavity surgery

Prewarming can be accomplished by:

- Providing a warm blanket
- Providing an insulated reflective blanket or head covering
- Ensuring an ambient room temperature of more than 73.4°F (23°C)
- Using a forced-air warming device (most widely used method)
- Warming intravenous fluids, blood, or blood products

Essential Facts

Question: You are taking care of an elderly, underweight patient with diabetes. What are some ways to prevent inadvertent perioperative hypothermia?

(continued)

(continued)

> **Answer:** Provide a warm blanket, use a forced-air warming device, make sure the room is at least 73°F, use a reflective blanket or head covering, and use warmed intravenous fluids, blood, or blood products.

Reference

Giuliano, K. K., & Hendricks, J. (2017). Inadvertent perioperative hypothermia: Current nursing knowledge. *AORN Journal*, *105*(5), 453–463.

3

Patient Positioning

The surgical team is responsible for positioning the patient for surgery to avoid undue injury to the patient and the surgical team. It is important to understand the goals of positioning, the physiologic effects of positioning, and the devices or equipment available to aid in positioning.

During this part of your orientation, you will learn about:

- Goals of positioning
- Risks for injury to the patient during positioning
- Types of positions
- Available devices and equipment to assist with positioning
- Use of ergonomics to protect yourself from injury

GENERAL CONSIDERATIONS FOR SAFE AND EFFECTIVE PATIENT POSITIONING

The overall goals of effectively positioning the patient are to:

- Prevent injury, skin breakdown, and nerve injury
- Maintain airway and pulmonary function
- Provide optimum surgical exposure

The following factors put patients at risk for injury due to positioning:

- Body weight extremes
- Poor nutritional status

- Diabetes
- Poor lifestyle choices (e.g., smoking)
- Elderly (> 70 years old)
- Peripheral vascular disease
- Hereditary peripheral neuropathy
- Anatomic variables (e.g., limited movement of a joint)
- Surgeries lasting longer than 4 hours

General safety guidelines for positioning are to:

- Provide adequate and optimum operative site exposure
- Make sure that there is access to intravenous and other monitoring equipment
- Check and recheck positioning throughout the surgical procedure
- Avoid undue pressure that can compromise circulation
- Use positioning devices according to the manufacturer's recommendations

Common positioning injuries are:

- Peripheral nerve stretching or pressure that can lead to transient or permanent nerve damage
- Skin breakdown from unrelieved pressure, duration of pressure, or patient's inability to withstand an increase in pressure

Essential Facts

Pressure as low as 23 to 32 mmHg can disrupt normal tissue. This exerts as little pressure as does placing a 1-inch cube weighing less than half a pound on a patient. Think about how little that really weighs and how little pressure it takes to cause injury to normal tissue.

SPECIAL CONSIDERATIONS FOR PROVIDING PATIENT PROTECTION FROM PRESSURE INJURIES

It is important to decrease pressure on any bony prominence. When positioning the patient, it is essential to have the devices available to protect the patient from any additional pressure and utilize these devices according to the individual patient needs. This can be accomplished by using:

- Gel products made of dry polymer elastomer gels
- Fluid-filled pads
- Pressure reduction and redistribution devices

STANDARD SURGICAL POSITIONS

There are many surgical positions, and they are dependent upon the type of surgery, the surgeon's preference, the anesthetic given, and the patient's limitations. The following sections cover some of the standard, more common surgical positions, and considerations necessary for a successful outcome.

Supine (Dorsal Recumbent)

- The patient lies on his or her back with either the arms on an arm board or tucked in at the side, if necessary (Figure 3.1). When the arm is extended on the arm board, the patient's palm should be facing up and the fingers should be extended. When the arm is tucked in at the side, the arm should be in a neutral position with the palm facing inward.

This is a common position for:

- Abdominal surgery
- Thoracic and cardiac surgery
- Neck and head surgery

Areas common for skin breakdown in the supine position are:

- Back of head
- Scapulae
- Elbows
- Vertebrae
- Sacrum

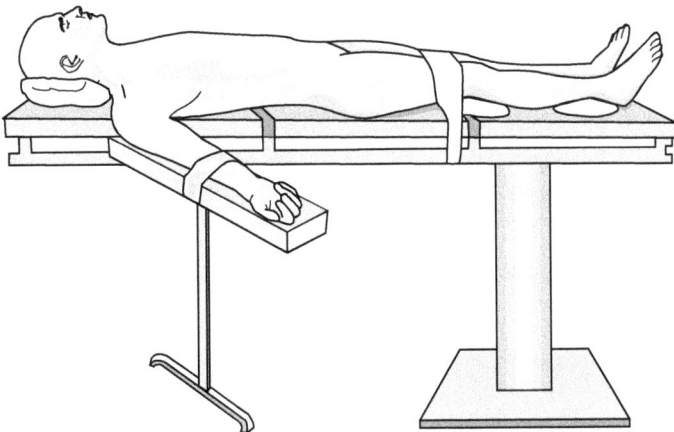

Figure 3.1 Supine position.

- Coccyx
- Heels

Nerves that can be injured in the supine position are:

- Brachial plexus
- Ulnar nerve

Positioning devices for the supine position:

- Safety belt secured about 2 inches above the knees
- Arm boards less than 90° abducted with palms facing up
- Wrist straps to secure arms on arm boards
- Head placed in a headrest

Essential Facts

Question: What devices and equipment should you have available for placing a patient in the supine position?
Answer: Safety belt, two arm boards, draw sheet, wrist straps, headrest, extra gel pads

Prone

The patient lies on his or her abdomen with either the arms on arm boards above the head or with the arms tucked at the sides, if necessary (Figure 3.2). This position can be exaggerated or modified into a jackknife (Kraske) position (Figure 3.3).

This is a common position for:

- Back surgery
- Rectal surgery

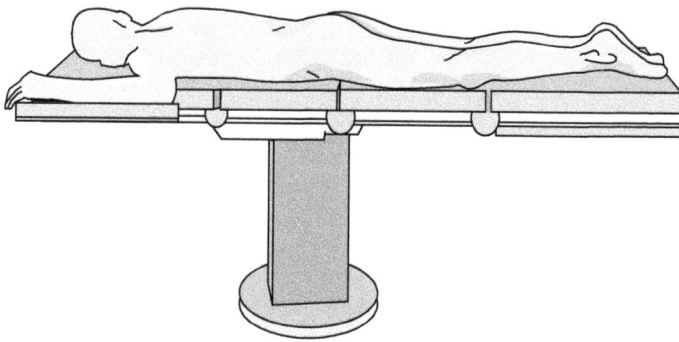

Figure 3.2 Prone position.

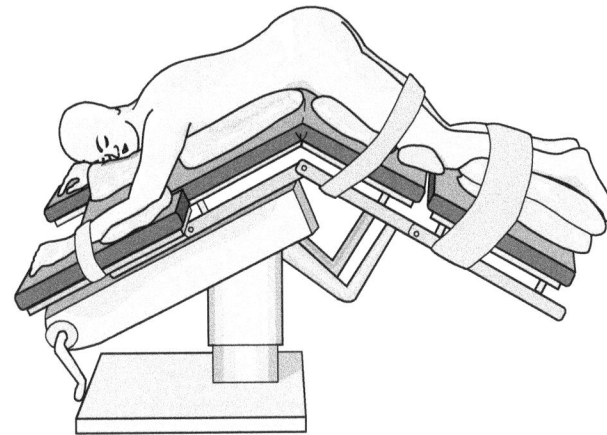

Figure 3.3 Kraske position.

Areas common for skin breakdown in the prone position are:

- Cheeks
- Eyes
- Ears
- Breasts
- Genitalia
- Patellas
- Toes

Nerve that can be injured in the prone position include:

- Brachial plexus

Positioning devices for the prone position:

- Safety belt secured approximately 2 inches above the back of the knees
- Arm boards less than 90° from shoulders with palms facing down
- Wrist straps to secure arms
- Head placed in a headrest

Other safety considerations for the prone position:

- Be aware of potential eye injury due to increased pressure.
- Support the chest and the pelvis to prevent pressure on the abdomen and compromised respirations.

Lithotomy

The patient begins in the supine position and the legs are raised and placed in stirrups (Figure 3.4). The arms can be positioned on arm boards or be tucked at the sides.

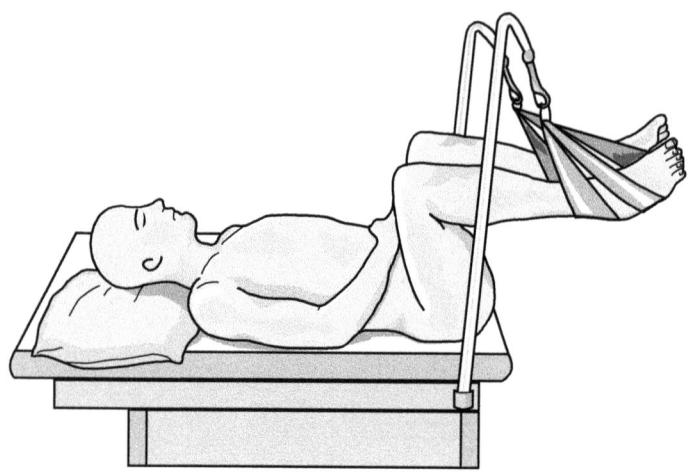

Figure 3.4 Lithotomy position.

Essential Facts

It is important to remember that if the arms must be tucked at the sides in the lithotomy position and when the break of the bed is elevated at the end of the surgery, then the fingers can be crushed. The fingers must be watched and protected!

This is a common position for:

- Gynecological surgery
- Rectal surgery
- Urological surgery

Areas common for skin breakdown in the lithotomy position are:

- Feet
- Ankles
- Knees

Nerves that can be injured in the lithotomy position are:

- Peroneal
- Sciatic
- Saphenous

Positioning devices for the lithotomy position:

- Safety belt secured approximately 2 inches above the back of the knees
- Arm boards less than 90° from shoulders with palms facing up

- Wrist straps to secure arms
- Head placed in headrest
- Stirrups
- Gel pad under sacrum

In the lithotomy position, types of stirrups used are dependent upon the type of surgery and the surgeon. They should be placed at even height. The legs should be lifted and lowered evenly and slowly into the stirrups. There are four levels of lithotomy:

- Low
- Standard
- High
- Exaggerated

Types of stirrups (Table 3.1) include:

- Ankle (candy-cane shape; Figure 3.5)
- Boot (Figure 3.6)
- Knee-crutch (Figure 3.7)

Lateral

The patient lies on the nonoperative side (Figure 3.8). When indicating laterality in this position, the dependent side that the patient is lying on is the reference point. Therefore, *left lateral* refers to when the patient lies on the left side.

It is important to consider that the patient's lower leg should be bent and the upper leg should be straight. Also, a pillow should be put between the legs, knees, ankles, and feet to avoid pressure. The upper arm should be secured on an arm board or padded surface with the

Table 3.1

Stirrup Considerations

Type of Stirrup	Positioning	Areas of Concern	Can Cause
Ankle	Secure foot in double sling and suspend.	Lateral aspect of calf and knee	Foot drop, nerve injury
Knee	Rest and secure leg on padded knee rest.	Popliteal space	Posterior peroneal nerve injury, popliteal artery
Boot	Rest and secure leg in padded boot.	Stress on hips	Hip, knee, leg injury; sciatic or obturator injury

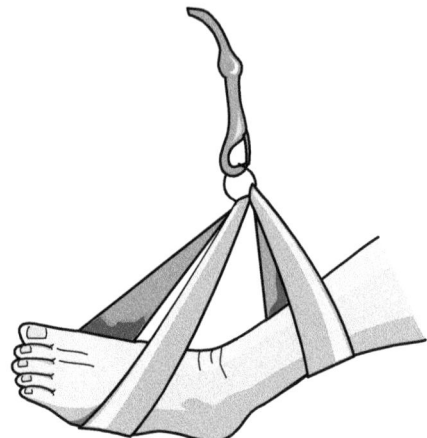

Figure 3.5 Ankle stirrup.

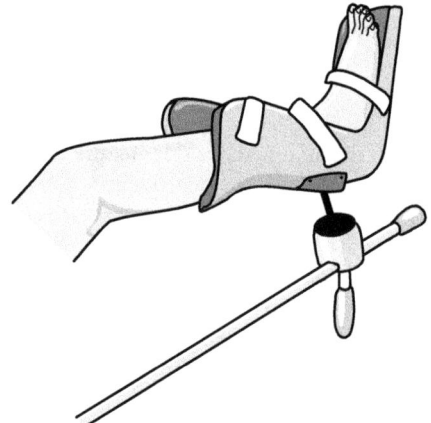

Figure 3.6 Boot stirrup.

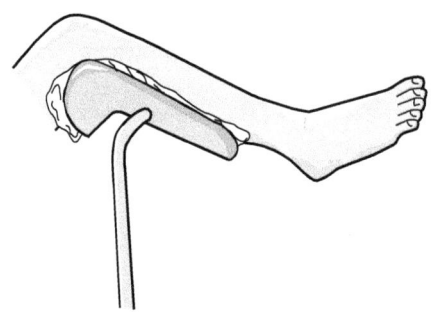

Figure 3.7 Knee-crutch stirrup.

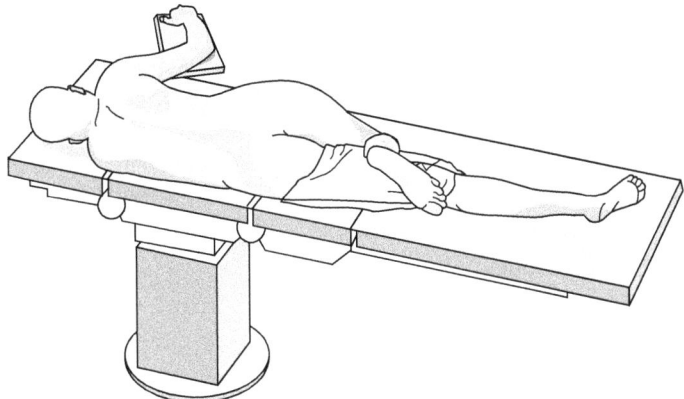

Figure 3.8 Lateral position.

palm down. The lower arm should be secured on a padded arm board with the palm up.

This is a common position for:

- Upper chest surgery
- Kidney surgery
- Hip surgery

Areas common for skin breakdown in the lateral position are:

- Elbows
- Ear
- Hip
- Lateral knee
- Ankle

Nerve that can be injured in the lateral position is:

- Peroneal nerve

Positioning devices for the lateral position are:

- Safety belt secured approximately 2 inches above the back of the knees
- Arm boards less than 90° from shoulders
- Wrist straps to secure arms
- Head placed on headrest
- Pillows
- Gel pad under body

Trendelenburg

The Trendelenburg position is also called the *shock position*. This is when the patient is in supine position and the bed is inverted, with the patient's head toward the floor and legs toward the ceiling (Figure 3.9). The knees of the patient may be bent to prevent the patient from sliding off of the operating room (OR) bed. Patients should remain in the Trendelenburg position for only as long as necessary. Respiratory exchange can be compromised, due to increased pressure on the diaphragm. Also, circulatory changes may occur in this position.

This is a common position for:

- Lower abdominal surgery
- Gynecological surgery
- Laparoscopic surgery

Areas common for skin breakdown in the Trendelenburg position are:

- Back of head
- Scapulae
- Elbows
- Vertebrae
- Sacrum
- Coccyx
- Heels

Nerves that can be injured in the Trendelenburg position include:

- Brachial plexus

Positioning devices for the Trendelenburg position are:

- Safety belt secured approximately 2 inches above the back of the knees

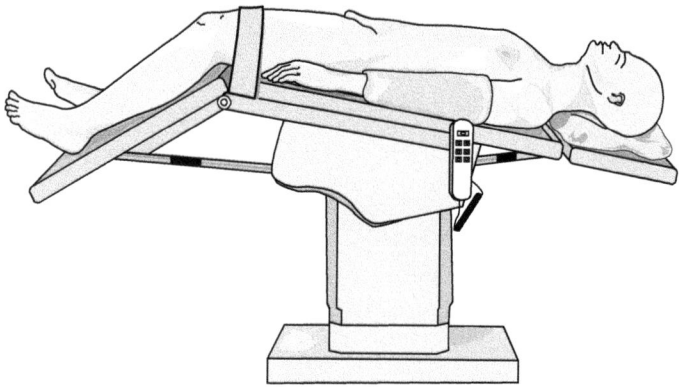

Figure 3.9 Trendelenburg position.

- Arm boards less than 90° from shoulders
- Wrist straps to secure arms
- Head placed on headrest

Note that shoulder braces should be avoided.

AN OUNCE OF PREVENTION: ADDITIONAL CONSIDERATIONS FOR PATIENT SAFETY

There are a few ways to prevent injury, skin breakdown, and nerve damage. This can be accomplished through a thorough nursing assessment and evaluation. It is important to:

- Identify tissue perfusion.
- Recognize sensory impairment.
- Detect musculoskeletal limitations.
- Discuss pain perception status.
- Evaluate peripheral pulses.
- Document variances.
- Suggest the use of a nerve conduction monitor on high-risk patients.

Not *all* cases of injury, skin breakdown, and nerve damage can be eliminated, but they can most definitely be minimized by proper assessment, planning, and interventions by the surgical team. It is important to continuously reassess the patient's position throughout the surgical procedure, especially when repositioning the patient or adjusting the OR bed. Also, always maintain dignity during positioning of the patient by exposing only the necessary area for the surgical procedure.

ERGONOMIC AND SAFETY CONSIDERATIONS FOR THE SURGICAL TEAM

It is important to protect yourself when positioning patients on the OR table for surgery. Therefore, here are a few tips to follow to keep yourself safe:

- Always solicit enough help.
- Communicate clearly so that lifting occurs simultaneously.
- Bend your knees when assisting during a lift.
- Stand as close to the OR bed as possible for leverage.
- Always utilize a lifting/transferring device, such as a lateral transfer device, an air-assisted lateral transfer device, or a

Table 3.2

Safe Patient Handling and Movement for Surgical Positions

Position	Patient Weight (Pounds)	Number of Personnel (People)	Transfer Device
Supine	<157	4	Lateral transfer device
	>157	3–4	Air-assisted lateral transfer device, mechanical lateral transfer device, or mechanical lift with supine sling
Prone	<73	2–4	Manual lifting
	>73	3–4	Mechanical lift preferred
Lithotomy	<141	2	Manual lifting
	>141	4	Use assistive device
Lateral	<115	4	Manual lifting
	>115	3	Use assistive device

Source: Adapted from Association of periOperative Registered Nurses Safe Patient Handling Pocket Reference Guide (2017).

mechanical lift depending on the weight of the patient and the desired position (Table 3.2).
- Make sure the transfer vehicle that the patient is being moved onto and the OR bed are both in the locked position.

Essential Facts

Question: The patient needs to be moved into the lateral position, but only you and the anesthesiologist are available. Should you move the patient into position?

Answer: No—you must solicit additional assistance, such as from the surgeon, resident, medical school student, and/or ancillary support. You must also obtain a lifting/transferring device to assist in moving the patient if the patient is over 115 pounds.

Reference

Association of periOperative Registered Nurses. (2017). AORN safe patient handling pocket reference guide. Retrieved from https://www.aorn.org/guidelines/clinical-resources/tool-kits/safe-patient-handling-tool-kit

4

Surgical Skin Preparation

The skin is the body's first line of defense. Although skin cannot be sterilized, it should be as clean as possible. Therefore, careful consideration must be given to choosing and using antiseptic agents as well as in properly preparing the skin for surgery.

During this part of your orientation, you will learn about:

- The goals and principles of skin preparation
- When to remove hair
- How to choose the best skin antiseptic
- Hazards of skin preparation

The goals of skin preparation are to:

- Remove soil, debris, exudate, and transient organisms from the surface of the skin.
- Decrease the risk of surgical-site infections (SSIs).
- Minimize the microbial count on the skin for a sustained period of time.

HAIR REMOVAL PRIOR TO SKIN PREPARATION

Over the years, hair removal has been a very controversial issue. Hair should be left in place whenever possible. If hair must be removed, use surgical clippers or depilatory creams, so that there is minimal injury to the skin. Razors are not recommended.

If hair must be removed, due to interference with the surgical procedure, hair removal should be:

- Performed the day of surgery
- Performed outside of the operating room unless an emergency
- Limited to as small an area as possible
- Removed with a single-use clipper or with a depilatory, if skin testing has been done first

SKIN INSPECTION

Once the hair has been addressed, the skin should be carefully inspected for:

- Rash
- Irritation
- Break in skin integrity

CHOOSING THE SKIN ANTISEPTIC AGENT

Choosing the correct antiseptic for skin is based on:

- Patient sensitivity or allergies
- Area being prepared
- Presence of open wounds or blood
- Surgeon's preference

The types of antiseptic agents to choose from are:

- Alcohol
- Chlorhexidine gluconate (CHG)
- Povidone–iodine
- CHG with alcohol
- Iodine-based with alcohol

The antiseptic agent used on skin must be approved by the U.S. Food and Drug Administration and must be used according to the manufacturer's directions and institutional policy and procedures. Antiseptic agents and their locations of use are listed in Table 4.1.

Essential Facts

Question: If you are preparing a neonate for surgery, which antiseptic agent would be your best choice?
Answer: Povidone–iodine used sparingly is the best choice.

Table 4.1

Antiseptic Agents and Locations of Use

Antiseptic Agent	Eyes	Ears	Mucous Membrane	Neonate
Alcohol	No	Yes	No	No
CHG	No	No	Yes, with caution	Safety not established
Povidone–iodine	Yes	Yes	Yes	Can cause iodism[a]
CHG with alcohol	No	No	No	No
Iodine based with alcohol	No	No	No	No

[a]Iodism is iodine poisoning.
CHG, chlorhexidine gluconate.

APPLICATION OF SKIN ANTISEPTIC AGENT

The application of the skin antiseptic agent should be performed by non-scrubbed personnel. This is because the risk of contamination is very high and it is important to keep the scrub nurse/surgical technologist sterile.

Basic principles for skin preparation:

- Wash and dry hands.
- Ask the anesthesia provider whether you can touch the patient.
- Identify and confirm the surgical site.
- Inspect the skin.
- Open up the skin preparation kit or applicator.
- Apply sterile gloves.
- Place sterile towels where the prep is being performed on the sides of the patient to absorb any residual antiseptic solution.
- Begin at the incision site and extend outward.
- Do not go over the same area; keep extending outward.
- Remember to remove the sterile towels at the end of the skin preparation.

Special considerations:

- Any contaminated area (e.g., rectum, vagina) should be prepared last.
- A stoma is prepped last, but a sponge soaked in antiseptic solution should be placed over the stoma initially, while doing the skin preparation.
- If the umbilicus is part of the skin preparation area, it should be cleaned first by using cotton-tipped applicators.

> **Essential Facts**
>
> Always communicate with the anesthesia provider before touching the surgical patient. During the immediate period after the induction of anesthesia, any sudden movement of the patient can cause a change in the patient's status (e.g., blood pressure, pulse, and laryngospasm). Therefore, it is important to indicate to the anesthesia provider that the skin preparation is going to begin.

HOW FAR YOU SHOULD GO?

There are general guidelines on how extensive a skin preparation should be, but this may vary according to:

- Surgeon preference
- Surgical procedure
- Individual patient

The prepped area should be extensive enough to accommodate:

- Drape shifting
- An extended incision
- An additional incision
- A change in procedure (e.g., laparoscopic to open approach)
- Possible drain-site access

> **Essential Facts**
>
> **Question:** If the surgeon indicates that he or she is performing a laparoscopic cholecystectomy, what part of the body should the nurse prepare?
> **Answer:** It is recommended that one prepares from the nipple line down to the middle of the thighs, in case the laparoscopy becomes an open abdominal procedure.

HAZARDS OF SKIN PREPARATION

There are four common hazards in skin preparation:

- Chemical burn
- Thermal burn

- Skin irritation
- Surgical flammability resulting in a potential fire

These hazards can be prevented by:

- Minimizing the use of antiseptic solution
- Cleaning up the dripping or pooling of antiseptic solution
- Using fluid-resistant towels to catch the solution
- Removing any linen with antiseptic solution residue
- Preventing solution from coming in contact with electrodes (e.g., EKG, electrosurgical unit ground pad)
- If using a pneumatic tourniquet, protect it from solution

Essential Facts

Flammable preparation agents must dry for the time specified by the manufacturer of the prep solution before draping the patient; otherwise, the alcohol vapor will accumulate under the drapes and can potentially ignite when using any heat source, such as electrocautery, laser, drill, or fiber optic.

At the end of any surgical procedure, the antiseptic agent should be removed from the skin, unless the manufacturer's directions note otherwise. This can prevent skin irritation and chemical burns. Some skin antiseptics, especially the alcohol-based variety, are made to remain on the skin postoperatively to maintain a persistent reduction in microorganisms on the skin surface. This will further help reduce SSIs.

5

Draping the Patient for Surgery

The surgical patient is draped prior to the commencement of the surgical procedure to create a sterile barrier between the surgical site and the rest of the operating room. This very important step will help prevent surgical-site infections (SSIs) and healthcare-associated infections.

During this part of your orientation, you will learn about:

- Different components of draping
- General principles of draping
- Potential problems associated with draping
- Removal of drapes at the conclusion of surgery

The overall goals of draping are to:

- Create and maintain a sterile field
- Prevent SSIs
- Minimize healthcare-associated infections

The Centers for Disease Control and Prevention recommends full-body draping for any procedure, including but not limited to those involving a peripherally inserted central catheter line, guide-wire exchange, and central venous catheter insertion.

COMPONENTS OF DRAPING

Drapes can be made of a woven fabric, which is usually reusable, or a nonwoven material that is disposable. Most draping materials are disposable. It is important for the scrub nurse or certified surgical technologist to stack the drapes, in the intended order of use, on the sterile field. This will make it easier to assist in the draping process. Each component is described as follows.

Towels

- Towels are made of woven cloth or paper with adhesive strips.
- Three or four towels are initially placed around the incision site.
- Towels may be held in place with staples, sutures, or nonperforated towel clips.

Sheet

- Commonly called *3/4 sheet*
- Comes in many sizes
- Covers anything that was left uncovered by the initial drapes
- Covers extremities
- Covers the feet if the fenestrated drape does not reach

Fenestrated Drape

- Commonly called *laparotomy (or lap) drape*
- Comes in various sizes for thyroid, breast, and chest surgery
- The incisional drape that covers the entire patient

Plastic Drape

- Commonly called iodophor-impregnated adhesive incise drape or *Vi-drape*
- Comes in many sizes
- Creates an impervious barrier, which means that fluid will not penetrate it
- Is resistant to fluid
- Is used when there is a high chance of irrigation and fluid loss
- Should not use adhesive incise drape without antimicrobial properties to prevent SSIs[1]

Stockinette

- Comes in many sizes
- Can be made of cloth or plastic
- Is used to drape an extremity when the extremity needs to freely move (e.g., as in hip or knee surgery)

---

[1] Evidence does not support the use of plastic adhesive incise drapes over incisions during surgical procedures to help limit infections. Research has found that this can actually increase infection rates.

Essential Facts

When opening the drapes from their original packaging onto the sterile field, the integrity of the package must be carefully examined. Inspect for holes, note expiration date (if applicable), and check sterilization indicators.

Before beginning the draping process, it is important to assess the quality of the skin and be certain that any solutions used in the skin preparation are completely dry. This will prevent the chance of surgical fire related to vapors accumulating under the drapes.

Choices of draping materials are dependent on:

- The procedure
- The size of the patient
- The patient position
- Surgeon preference
- Available products at your organization

BASIC PRINCIPLES OF DRAPING

- When walking with drapes, keep them folded and close to your body at waist height.
- Handle drapes as little as possible.
- Do not shake out or wave drapes.
- Always hold drapes above the height of the operating room table and bed.
- Draping starts at the incision site and moves outward.
- Drape nearest to farthest to prevent reaching over unsterile areas.
- Do not reposition or move drapes after placement.
- If drapes become contaminated, discard as soon as feasible.
- Cuff hands when draping to protect from contaminating with unsterile areas.[2]

Essential Facts

Excessive movement of drapes can create air currents and propel dust, lint, and other contaminating particles into the air, which can land on the sterile field or in a patient's incision.

---

[2] *Cuff hands* means that the drape completely covers the gloved hand so that the hand does not touch anything that is not sterile. The scrub nurse wraps the drape securely around the gloved hand, as in Figure 5.1.

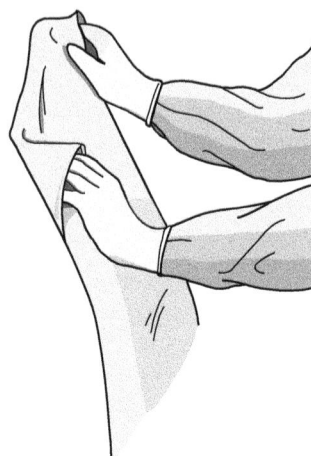

Figure 5.1 Cuffed sterile hand in drape.

- Look for tears or holes in drapes.
- If a drape becomes torn, it must be covered with another sterile drape.

COMMON ORDER OF DRAPES FOR A BASIC SURGERY

All surgeries, surgeons, and organizations will have specific guidelines to follow when draping a patient for surgery, but this is the common order in which drapes would be placed:
- Four towels
- Fenestrated drape (i.e., lap drape)
- Additional sheet

It is quite common to have to secure items to the drapes. These items include:

- Suction tubing
- Electrocautery devices
- Other energy devices
- Smoke-evacuator tubing

SECURING ITEMS TO THE DRAPES

- Use blunt towel clips to prevent perforation of drape material.
- Use fenestrated premade holes to hold tubing.

- Use plastic instrument pouches that attach with adhesive to hold surgical devices securely.
- Use velcro tube/line holders that attach to drapes with adhesive or come premade on drapes.
- Use plastic pouches that can be attached to the drape and catch excess fluid or irrigation (e.g., as in a cesarean section).

STRIKE-THROUGH: AN IMPORTANT INFECTION CONTROL CONSIDERATION

If the drape material becomes moist and permeated, this is considered "strike-through." When this happens, bacteria can migrate up and onto the sterile field. The drape is considered contaminated and must be covered or changed. Strike-through is more common with cloth drapes, but paper draping material can also become permeated during surgeries that have a copious amount of irrigation fluid or blood loss. It is important to always be looking for strike-through.

REMOVAL OF DRAPES

At the end of the surgical procedure, the drapes must be removed by:

- First covering the incision with sterile dressing
- Carefully removing surrounding drapes by rolling them onto themselves
- Wearing gown, gloves, and eye protection to prevent contamination
- Disposing in the proper receptacle

Essential Facts

Question: What do you do if you take off your gown, gloves, and personal protective equipment and are then asked to assist in taking off the drapes?
Answer: You must put on a gown, gloves, and eye protection before you assist in taking off the drapes. A shortcut of just putting utility gloves on is easy, but exposes you to potential contamination by blood and body fluids and creates an unsafe situation.

DRAPING OTHER ITEMS IN THE OPERATING ROOM

Besides the patient, there are other items in the operating room that require draping. These items include:

- Equipment (e.g., microscope, x-ray machine)
- Furniture (e.g., Mayo stand)
- Table parts adjacent to the sterile field

These items must be draped so that the scrubbed personnel can handle them safely. It is important to follow the same basic principles that apply to draping a surgical patient. Also, once draped, these items should remain as close to the sterile field as possible in order to avoid contamination.

LEAD APRONS

Whenever an x-ray or fluoroscopy (continuous x-ray) is being used, a lead apron should be worn by each member of the surgical team to protect him or her from radiation. The lead apron should be donned prior to scrubbing, gowning, and gloving. It should be accompanied by a thyroid shield, which is a small lead shield that goes around the neck to cover the thyroid gland. The thyroid gland is one of the most radiosensitive organs in the body, and exposure to radiation can contribute to thyroid cancer. Leaded eyeglasses with side shields are also recommended to be worn by personnel, who are close to the radiation, especially during fluoroscopic procedures, in order to prevent injury to the eyes. Sterile radiation-attenuated gloves should be worn by scrub personnel whose hands will be in line with the direct radiation beam.

Important considerations of lead aprons include:

- Maintain the integrity of the apron by avoiding folding the apron, and by hanging aprons on racks when not in use.
- Be certain to choose the appropriate-sized lead apron, so that it covers long bones of the upper portion of the legs and is inclusive of the upper chest, specifically the breast area.
- Wrap the apron around the body to cover as much of the body as possible, to prevent radiation exposure.
- Inspect aprons annually using fluoroscopic or radiographic examination to identify cracks or holes in the lead.
- Clean aprons after each use.

RADIATION BADGE (THERMOLUMINESCENT DOSIMETER)

Many institutions require members of the surgical team to wear a radiation badge due to their frequent exposure to radiation. This badge is worn on the outside of the lead apron when participating in any procedures that require x-rays or fluoroscopy. The badges must be monitored and reported according to the radiation protocol of the institution.

II

Environment and Processing Considerations

6

Operating Room Environment Requirements

The operating room environment must be clean and safe for the patient and the perioperative team. It is important to utilize the proper cleaning supplies, control the environmental conditions, and understand infectious processes that can potentially transmit harmful microorganisms into the operating room environment.

During this part of your orientation, you will learn about:

- The requirements of properly cleaning the operating room
- The temperature, airflow, humidity, and air-exchange requirements
- Traffic patterns
- Different types of patient precautions related to infection control

CLEANING THE OPERATING ROOM ENVIRONMENT

The products used to clean the operating room must be registered with the Environmental Protection Agency (EPA) and contain chemicals that are appropriate for all patient populations. These products must also remove soil, debris, and blood products.

These products contain

- A detergent that cleans debris from the surface
- A disinfectant that decreases the viral and bacterial count on the surface

These products can be

- One step, meaning that they contain both a detergent and a disinfectant in one product
- Two step, meaning that each product is used individually

It is important to remember that disinfectants must remain on a surface for a specific contact time to be effective. The amount of time is specific to the product and the product must be used within the manufacturer's recommendations. Also, disinfectant does not sterilize a surface. Disinfectants only decrease the presence of pathogens.

Properties of a disinfectant:

- Broad spectrum (works on a wide range of microorganisms)
- Fast acting
- Nontoxic
- Compatible with different surfaces
- Has an antimicrobial residual effect
- Easy to use
- Cost-effective
- Environmentally friendly

Types of disinfectants:

- Phenolics
- Quaternary ammonium compounds
- Iodophors
- Chlorine (bleach)

The type of disinfectant is dependent upon the type of surface and the infectious material on the surface.

ALCOHOL

Alcohol should never be used to disinfect environmental surfaces because it is not an EPA-registered disinfectant. It is important to remember that alcohol does not remove soil from a surface and is also very flammable.

ASSESSING THE OPERATING ROOM ENVIRONMENT

The RN, certified surgical technologist, and any member of the perioperative team should continually assess the environment for cleanliness. This can be accomplished through:

- Visual inspection for soil, dirt, or organic matter
- Damp dusting (wiping all horizontal surfaces with an appropriate disinfectant) at the start of the day before any instruments, supplies, or equipment are moved into the room

Essential Facts

Any item that lands on the floor is considered contaminated and needs to be either disinfected or discarded.

Items that need to be cleaned after each use are high-touch items, such as:

- Operating room bed, remote control, safety belt
- Positioning devices
- Carts
- Intravenous (IV) poles
- Monitors and control panel
- Tables
- Equipment
- Knobs, switches, and handles

Items that need to be cleaned *only when visibly soiled* include:

- Floor
- Walls

Each day that the operating room is in use, it should be terminally cleaned. This means that at the end of the day, the operating room should be completely wiped down.

Terminal cleaning includes removal of all trash and cleaning the following items:

- Floors after the last procedure of the day
- All exposed surfaces
- Equipment
- Wheels of any carts, tables, or equipment
- Handles of cabinets and doors
- Ventilation plates

Essential Facts

Question: Upon the removal of the drapes, some blood and body fluid drips onto the operating room floor. When does this need to be cleaned up?

Answer: Floors need to be cleaned after each surgical procedure, if soiled or potentially soiled. Therefore, upon the completion of the surgery, the floor must be cleaned. Also, an absorbent towel should be placed over the spill to contain it and to keep the perioperative personnel safe from slipping.

TEMPERATURE, AIRFLOW, HUMIDITY, AND AIR EXCHANGE

These environmental considerations should be continuously monitored and recorded. This will ensure comfort for the staff and patient, an optimum aseptic environment, safety, and control of smells (Figure 6.1).

Essential Facts

If humidity is too high, supplies will become damp/moist, which can increase growth of microorganisms. If humidity is too low, dust and static electricity are increased. This can increase the chance of surgical-site infections and the chance of fires.

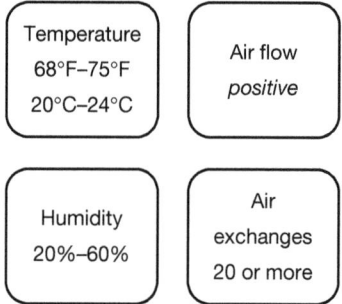

Figure 6.1 Temperature, airflow, humidity, and air exchange (Association of periOperative Registered Nurses, 2017) (ANSI/ASHRAE/ASHE Standard 170-2017 Design Perameters, Hospital Spaces)

TRAFFIC PATTERNS

Traffic patterns vary depending upon the logistics of each organization, but all should consider the following:

- Patient privacy
- Safety of everyone
- Security of supplies and equipment

The operating room is a restricted area, but it still must abide by strict rules to help maintain these considerations. These include:

- Maintain a clear separation between clean and dirty supplies and equipment.
- Keep movement and activity in and out of the room to a minimum, due to shedding of microbes.
- Keep doors closed to maintain air pressure, air exchanges, temperature, and humidity.
- Keep the number of people in the operating room to a minimum.
- Keep talking to a minimum.

TRANSMISSION-BASED PRECAUTIONS

Patients are subjected to different types of precautions depending on the etiology of their disease. These can include:

- Standard precautions
- Contact precautions
- Droplet precautions
- Airborne precautions

Standard Precautions

All members of the perioperative team should abide by the general standard precautions in the operating room. This will help prevent the transmission of infectious diseases. This can be accomplished by:

- Proper hand hygiene between patients and when hands are visibly soiled
- Use of personal protective equipment (PPE) when there is possible exposure to blood or body fluids (i.e., mask, eye protection, gloves, cover jacket, gown)
- Proper and up-to-date personal immunization (e.g., hepatitis B vaccine)

Contact Precautions

Providing care to any patient who may have an infectious process that can be transmitted through direct contact requires contact precautions. It is important to follow these rules:

- Use PPE (mask, gloves, eye protection, gown).
- Wash with soap and water, if in direct contact with blood or body fluids.
- If transporting patient, cover patient's affected area.
- Clearly communicate with caregivers that the patient is on contact precautions.

Some infectious disease processes that require contact precautions include:

- Multiple-drug-resistant organisms (MDROs), which refers to any bacteria resistant to antibiotic therapy
- Methicillin-resistant *Staphylococcus aureus* (MRSA)
- Vancomycin-resistant enterococci (VRE)
- *Clostridium difficile*

Droplet Precautions

When providing care to any patient who may have an infectious disease process that is transmitted through large droplets (5 or more microns) that can be inhaled, it is important to follow these rules:

- Use PPE if within 3 feet of the patient.
- The patient should wear a mask during transport.
- Clearly communicate with caregivers that the patient is on droplet precautions.

Some infectious disease processes that require droplet precautions include:

- COVID-19
- Influenza (flu)
- Pertussis
- Fifth disease

Airborne Precautions

When providing care to any patient who may have an infectious disease process that is transmitted through small droplets (less than 5 microns) that can be inhaled, it is important to follow these rules:

- Use PPE, including an N95 respirator.
- Use an isolation room that has a special air-exchange and ventilation system with negative pressure.
- If transporting the patient, cover the patient's nose and mouth with a mask.
- Clearly communicate with caregivers that the patient is on airborne precautions.
- Go directly to the operating room and do not bring the patient to areas with other patients.

Some infectious disease processes that require airborne precautions include:

- Tuberculosis
- Rubeola (measles)

- Varicella (chicken pox)
- COVID-19

CLEANING AFTER INFECTION-CONTROL PRECAUTIONS

Cleaning will vary depending upon the type of disease process the patient acquired. MDROs, such as MRSA and VRE, require a broad-spectrum disinfectant, whereas *Clostridium difficile* requires a 10% bleach solution.

Essential Facts

Question: Mr. Estevez is scheduled to come to the operating room for an emergent laparoscopic appendectomy. The nurse from the emergency department indicated that he is on "droplet precautions." What considerations should be made?

Answer: Mr. Estevez should wear a mask when being transported and any caregiver within 3 feet should also have PPE on, which includes a mask, eye protection, and gloves. A gown should be worn if necessary depending upon what needs to be done to the patient.

NOISE IN THE OPERATING ROOM

There is a great deal of ambient background noise in the operating room. Some examples of this include:
- Monitors
- Talking
- Equipment (drills, smoke evacuator)
- Environment (heating, ventilation, and air-conditioning [HVAC] system)
- Cell phones
- Music

It is important to try to minimize the excess ambient noise to effectively communicate, think critically, and hear the clinical alarms.

Some helpful hints are:

- Lubricate doors and wheels.
- Limit unnecessary people in the operating room.
- Discourage phones and beepers in the ring mode.

- Set alarms at appropriate auditory levels.
- Limit overhead pages and announcements.
- Improve awareness through education.

WASTE DISPOSAL

Everything that is used in the operating room has to go somewhere. Depending on the item, the waste disposal will vary.

Items fall into different categories:

- Noncontaminated (e.g., packaging materials) waste gets packaged as noninfectious waste.
- Infected (came in contact with blood or body fluids) waste goes in a closable and leak-resistant bag.
- Sharp objects (e.g., knife blade, needle) go in color-coded hard plastic boxes.
- Liquids require a solidifying powder that is then treated as infected waste or placed in a special medical liquid system.
- Pharmaceuticals require color-coded disposal bins used to separate hazardous from nonhazardous pharmaceutical wastes, based upon the U.S. EPA enforcement determined by each particular state's regulations.

Many organizations now consider recycling as an environmental responsibility. Also, many companies are making items that are partially reusable and contain fewer disposable materials. This helps contain costs and reduces waste.

Reference

Association of periOperative Registered Nurses. (2017). AORN safe patient handling pocket reference guide. Retrieved from https://www.aorn.org/guidelines/clinical-resources/tool-kits/safe-patient-handling-tool-kit

ANSI/ASHRAE/ASHE Standard 170-2017 Design Paramets, Hospital Spaces

7

Sterile Technique

The use of sterile technique ensures the protection of patients and prevents the perioperative personnel from acquiring or spreading infections. This reduces the chance of surgical-site infections. Hand washing is always the number one way to prevent the spread of infections, but sterile technique must be implemented and maintained to ensure positive patient outcomes.

During this part of your orientation, you will learn about:

- General principles of sterile technique
- Preparing the operating room for surgery
- Sterile packaging and how to handle each type
- Scrubbing, gowning, and gloving
- Setting up, maintaining, and breaking down the sterile field

Sterile means the absence of microorganisms, and therefore sterile technique involves the principles and procedures used to maintain an area free from microorganisms.

GENERAL PRINCIPLES OF STERILE TECHNIQUE

- Only sterile items can be used on the sterile field.
- Items that may not be sterile should automatically be presumed unsterile.

- Whenever a sterile field is compromised, it is considered contaminated.
- Only the top surface of a drape is considered sterile.
- The edges of a sterile-item's package are considered unsterile.
- Personnel who are gowned and considered sterile can only touch things that are also sterile.
- The patient is the center of the sterile field.

PREPARING THE OPERATING ROOM FOR SURGERY

The operating room is prepared for surgery by the circulating/scrubbing RN, the certified surgical technologist (CST), and the anesthesia provider. Each person has specific and complementary roles in acquiring and anticipating everything necessary to perform surgery. The better prepared, the less time the circulating nurse needs to leave the operating room during the procedure. As you will see, many of the roles overlap and can be performed by any member of the perioperative team. Therefore, effective communication is essential.

Role of the circulating nurse:

- Check inventory of necessary supplies
- Check functionality of equipment.
- Check integrity of sterile packaging.
- Open up supplies and equipment.
- Obtain and prepare any medications.
- Assess and educate the patient.
- Communicate with the perioperative team.

Role of the scrub nurse or CST:

- Check inventory of necessary supplies.
- Check functionality of equipment.
- Check integrity of sterile packaging.
- Open up supplies and equipment.
- Communicate with the perioperative team.
- Scrub, set up, and maintain the sterile field.
- Obtain and prepare any medications.

Role of the anesthesia provider:

- Check inventory of necessary supplies.
- Check functionality of anesthesia equipment.
- Obtain and prepare any medications.
- Assess and discuss anesthetic plan of care with patient/nurse.
- Communicate with the perioperative team.

DETERMINING STERILITY OF ITEMS

Before opening the sterile supplies, determine whether each item is sterile. This is a very important step because if something is not sterile, then the entire sterile field will be compromised and immediately considered unsterile.

Examine the integrity of the package:

- Check for holes.
- Check date of expiration, if applicable.
- Check for any discoloration.
- Check chemical indicator(s).

The date of expiration is most often an event-related item. This means that a date is not placed on an item, but an event must occur to render the package unsterile. Such events could be:

- Excessive handling that compromises the integrity of the package
- Moisture penetration
- Exposure to airborne contamination
- Temperature and humidity out of acceptable range

Chemical indicators are part of the monitoring process for sterilization. They determine whether the physical conditions of sterilization were met. This does not prove that the item is necessarily sterile, only that the conditions were met. More about the sterilization process will be discussed in the next chapter.

Essential Facts

Question: After careful examination of a sterile package, you notice that the chemical indicator did not change. What should you do?
Answer: Consider the item unsterile and do not open onto the sterile field. This item did not meet the physical conditions of sterilization.

TYPES OF STERILE SUPPLY PACKAGING

Sterile supplies come in many different sizes and types. Some such types are:

- Peel-and-seal pouch/bag (Figure 7.1)
- Envelope-style wrap (Figure 7.2)
- Manufacturer wrap

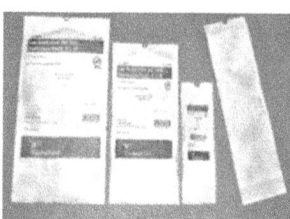

Figure 7.1 Peel-and-seal wrapper.

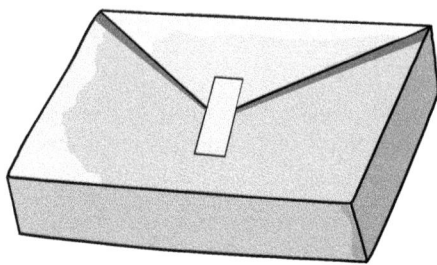

Figure 7.2 Envelope-style wrapper.

Opening each type of sterile supply packaging takes careful consideration and practice to ensure that the sterile item is delivered to the sterile field in a sterile condition.

Opening a peel-and-seal package:

- Inspect integrity.
- Gently peel back packaging from the angled edge.
- The edges are considered unsterile.
- The item should be presented to the scrubbed personnel directly or safely tossed onto the sterile field.

Opening envelope-style wrapper:

- Inspect integrity.
- Determine that the chemical indicator changed.
- Grasp in nondominant hand.
- With the dominant hand, open outward all four flaps (the furthest should be opened first, then sides, and then nearest).
- The edges are considered unsterile.
- Do not reach over the sterile item with an unsterile hand/arm.
- Grasp all three flaps with the dominant hand.
- The item should be presented to the scrubbed personnel directly or safely tossed onto the field.

Opening manufacturer's wrapper:

- Inspect integrity.
- Read packaging and determine sterility of item.

- Tear open at perforation.
- Take out the inner wrapper.
- Proceed with the last six steps for the envelope-style wrapper.

BASIC TECHNIQUE FOR DELIVERING ITEMS ONTO THE STERILE FIELD

The optimal way to present an item onto the sterile field is to hand it directly to the scrubbed personnel. This prevents the chance of the item rolling off the sterile field, displacing another item from the sterile field, or penetrating the sterile field due to the item being sharp or heavy.

TYPES OF STERILE INSTRUMENT PACKAGING

Opening sterile instrument packaging takes careful consideration and practice to ensure that the item is delivered to the sterile field with sterility intact. Instruments may be in different types of packaging:

- Peel-and-seal
- Envelope-style wrap
- Rigid sterilization container (canister)

The peel-and-seal and envelope-style wraps should be opened as described earlier for sterile supply packaging.

The rigid sterilization container (Figure 7.3) should be opened as follows:

- Place on a clean, flat, dry surface that is the height of the sterile field.
- Check that external locks are intact.
- Check external chemical indicator.
- Unlatch and lift upward toward self.
- Check filter(s) for integrity.
- If the container has more than one filter, each filter must be checked for holes; if holes are found, the tray is considered unsterile.
- Check internal chemical indicator(s).

SCRUBBING, GOWNING, AND GLOVING

The scrub nurse or CST will scrub, gown, and glove to set up the sterile field. It is important to remember to open a gown and gloves prior to going to the scrub sink to scrub. It is also recommended to place the sterile opened gown and gloves close to the sterile field, but not

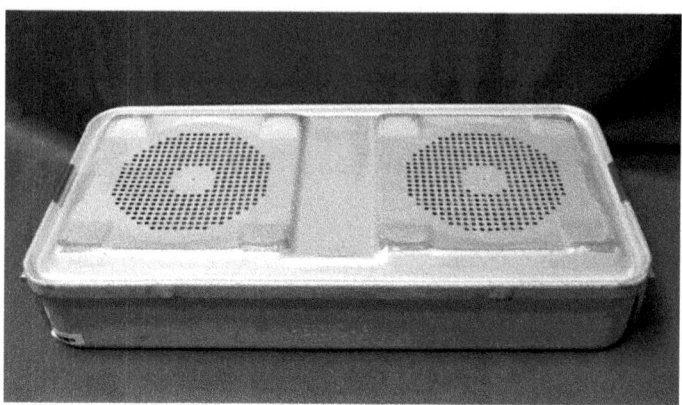

Figure 7.3 Rigid sterilization container.

on the sterile field. This will prevent the contamination of the sterile field with the unsterile arm when picking up the gown.

Scrub Soap Choices

The person scrubbing has two choices of soap to use—either an alcohol-based hand rub (Figure 7.4) or a scrub brush that is impregnated with an antimicrobial soap (Figure 7.5). Evidence in the literature supports the efficacy of the alcohol-based hand rub as the preferred method, but due to allergies and preferences, the scrub-brush method is still available and widely used.

Various types of scrub soaps can be:

- 1% chlorhexidine gluconate and 61% ethyl alcohol
- 4% chlorhexidine soap on a sterile scrub brush
- 7.5% povidone–iodine on a sterile scrub brush

Hand-rub technique:

- Remove all jewelry and watches.
- Clean under nails, wash hands with soap, and dry hands to remove transient flora (the bacteria that accumulates on the skin surface).
- Apply surgical hand rub according to manufacturer's recommendations.
- The product should be applied to the fingertips and hands, extending upward 2 inches above the elbow.
- Repeat on opposing hand and arm.
- Then the hands should be done again.
- The skin surface should air dry before gowning and gloving, which can take up to 90 seconds.

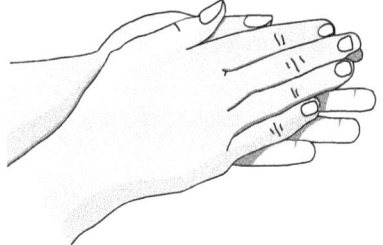

Figure 7.4 Hand rub.

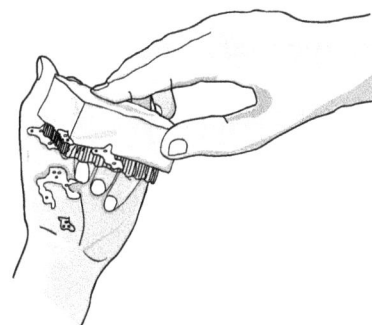

Figure 7.5 Hand scrub.

Scrub-brush technique:

- Remove all jewelry and watches.
- Wash hands with soap and dry hands to remove transient flora.
- Use a nail pick to clean under the nails.
- Use an impregnated scrub brush to brush fingertips, fingers, and hands on all four sides.
- Rinse brush and with sponge side proceed upward on the arm one third at a time on all four sides of the arm to 2 inches above the elbow.
- Rinse brush and proceed to the other arm.
- Time of application should be dictated according to manufacturer's directions.
- Discard scrub brush.
- Rinse each hand and arm from fingertip to 2 inches above the elbow without the water dripping downward onto the hands.

Gowning

The next step is to enter the operating room by using your back to open the door and keeping your hands elevated above waist height and at a 90° angle from your body. It is also important not to drip the water from your arms onto the sterile field that was created when you opened your gown and gloves.

- Lean forward and pick up the sterile towel (if the brush method was used) and pat dry from fingertips to 2 inches above the elbow; otherwise, proceed to next step.
- Carefully pick up the gown and open it with the arms facing outward, visualizing the arm holes and inner neckline facing you.
- Slide your arms into the gown until your hands are just about up to the cuff.
- Do not touch the outside of the gown.
- The circulating nurse will adjust the gown above the shoulders and clasp the back of the gown at the neck and the waist.
- Perform closed glove technique.
- The scrub will "tie in" by passing the paper tag to the circulating nurse and turning, then tying the strings to secure the gown at the waist.
- The wrist of the cuff of the gown must be covered by the glove at all times due to the fact that the wrist section is not impervious and is porous.

Closed-Glove Technique

One technique used to apply the sterile gloves after you put your gown on is called the *closed-glove technique* (Figure 7.6) and involves the following steps:

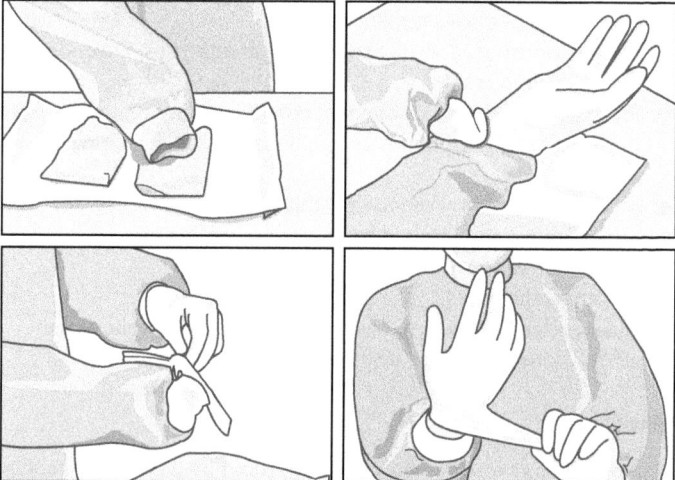

Figure 7.6 Closed-glove technique.

- Use the cuffed hands to open up the sterile glove paper by opening it like a book, grabbing the lower corners, and lifting them simultaneously outward.
- Take the dominant hand with palm up while using the opposing hand to place the glove on the dominant hand with the thumb-side down; glove fingers will point to your body.
- Grab the upper cuff of the glove with the opposing hand while holding the other side of the cuff through the gown with the dominant hand.
- Pull the glove over the cuff and wiggle fingers into the glove.
- Using the gloved hand, pick up the second glove and place it against the palm of the hand that is in the gown sleeve.
- Grab the cuff through the gown with the gloved hand while pulling it over the cuff.
- Adjust the fingers of both hands into the glove and pull the glove cuff over the gown cuff completely.
- Hand the paper tag from the gown to the circulating nurse.
- Turn and tie gown at the waist.

Most institutions recommend wearing two pairs of sterile gloves. This practice can prevent the possibility of a microscopic perforation in the glove contaminating your skin or the possibility of glove failure if stuck with a needle. It is also common to wear a darker colored underglove which makes it easier to identify a perforation.

Essential Facts

The act of double gloving can reduce the risk of exposure to patient blood by as much as 87% when the outer glove is punctured. The amount of blood on a solid suture needle is reduced by approximately 95% when it has to pass through two layers of glove.

Parts of the scrub personnel that are considered sterile are:

- Front of gown from 2 inches above the elbow to fingertips
- Below nipple line over to the axilla
- Above the waist at the height of the sterile field

Parts of the scrub personnel that are *not* considered sterile are:

- Neckline
- Shoulders
- Underarms
- Sleeve cuff
- Back of gown

SETTING UP AND MAINTAINING THE STERILE FIELD

There are some basic principles to adhere to when setting up and maintaining the sterile field:

- Only sterile items can be put on the sterile field.
- The sterile field must always be monitored.
- Do not reach over a sterile field unless sterile (gowned and gloved).
- Sterile personnel should not reach over unsterile areas.
- Movement around the sterile field should be limited.
- Sterility on the sterile field is only the table top to the edge of the table.
- If the drape does not cover the entire surface (i.e., gown wrapper), a 1-inch margin around the edge of the wrapper is not considered sterile.
- The outer edge of any heat-sealed wrapper is not considered sterile. Only the inner edge is sterile.
- Heavy or cumbersome items should not be "tossed" onto the sterile field but taken by the scrubbed personnel.
- Items should be opened as close to the time of surgery as possible. This will decrease the chance of contamination by particles in the air that can land on the sterile field.
- Handle supplies as little as possible.
- Large packs or equipment should be opened on a flat surface at the height of the sterile field.
- Once the patient enters the operating room, opened sterile supplies can only be used for that particular patient.

Essential Facts

Question: The patient is scheduled for surgery at 8 a.m., but is delayed until 10:30 a.m. Both the circulator and scrub would like to take a break to eat breakfast. What should they do?

Answer: Because the sterile field is opened, it must be continuously monitored. Therefore, one person must remain in the operating room observing that the sterile field is not being compromised. The circulator and scrub must take separate breaks to eat, while one remains with the sterile field.

TRANSFERRING ITEMS TO THE STERILE FIELD DURING THE SURGERY

Each item that needs to be transferred to the sterile field should first be inspected for its integrity and expiration, if applicable. Many times during a surgical procedure, additional items need to be passed onto the sterile field.

Options for solid items being transferred to the sterile field:

- The circulating nurse opens the item and the scrub personnel removes it from the wrapper with gloved hand or forceps.
- Tossing onto the field is discouraged due to the air turbulence and potential for contamination by dropping the item.
- The item is opened on a separate table by the circulator and taken by the scrub personnel.

Options for liquid items being transferred to the sterile field:

- The sterile container should be placed close to the edge of the sterile field in anticipation of pouring.
- The circulator pours into the sterile container, not reaching over the sterile field.
- Liquid must be labeled immediately by the scrubbed personnel.
- Re-capping of a container by the circulator is not recommended due to contamination during the action of pouring.

BREAKING DOWN THE STERILE FIELD

At the end of the surgical procedure, the sterile field is disassembled and the instruments are brought to the dirty workroom for processing.

The steps that should be taken are:

- Dispose of any sharp items in proper receptacles.
- Suction up any liquids on the field into the suction canisters or dispose of in proper receptacles.
- Place all instruments back in instrument containers.
- Dispose of any additional items, such as suctions, sponges, drapes, and so forth, in the proper receptacles.

Removal of Gown and Gloves

The removal of your gown and gloves (Figure 7.7) occurs after everything is cleaned up and disposed of. The gown and gloves protect you

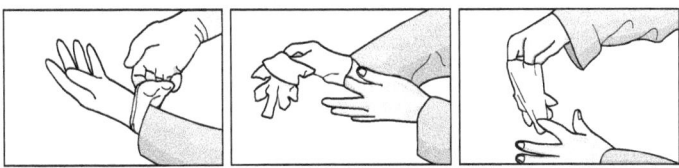

Figure 7.7 Removal of gloves.

from anything spilling on you as you dispose of liquids, drapes, and other items.

- Take off outer pair of gloves.
- Pull gown from the front and break the tie and neck clasp or have a nonscrubbed personnel untie and unclasp the gown.
- Pull gown over and off of body and arms.
- Remove gloves by only touching the outside of them with your gloved hand and then take your clean hand and reach into the opposing glove to pull off.
- Place dirty gown and gloves in proper receptacle.

Essential Facts

A simple way to remember how to unglove safely is "glove to glove, skin to skin." This means that the glove touches the glove while taking off the first glove and your ungloved hand touches the inside of the glove on your hand to remove the second glove.

8

Sterilization and Central Processing

All instrumentation and equipment used during a surgical procedure that are not disposable must go through a stringent process in order to be sterilized for reuse (Figure 8.1).

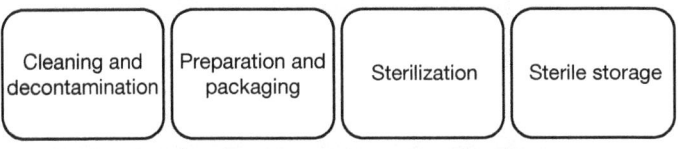

Figure 8.1 Sterilization process.

During this part of your orientation, you will learn about:

1. The components of each sterilization process
2. Different types of sterilization
3. Parameters of each type of sterilization
4. Advantages and disadvantages of each type of sterilization

CLEANING AND DECONTAMINATION

Upon the completion of surgery, all instrumentation and equipment from the sterile field must be prepared to be decontaminated before being sterilized for use. During this process, all personnel involved must protect themselves from blood or body fluids by wearing personal protective equipment, such as:

- Head covering
- Gown
- Gloves
- Mask with eye protection
- Shoe covers

Preparing the instruments and equipment for decontamination involves:

- Wiping off blood or debris with water because if not wiped it will dry and be more difficult to remove
- Opening instruments so box locks are exposed
- Flushing lumens or cannulated instruments
- Placing sharp instruments together, facing downward
- Disassembling instruments that have multiple parts
- Remove any disposable parts from instrumentation and discard
- Preventing the placement of heavy instruments on top of delicate instruments
- Placing cameras, scopes, and cords in their canisters
- Ensure instruments are kept wet by spraying with enzymatic solution

Essential Facts

It is important to remember not to use saline on instruments or equipment. The salt in the saline solution will rust or pit the instruments. Surgical instruments and equipment are very expensive and delicate, and must be treated with the utmost care.

Enzymatic Solution

Enzymatic solution will soften the dried blood or debris on instruments, resulting in much easier removal. Enzymatic cleaners can be liquid or come in a gel spray, which is very convenient and easy to apply to the instruments. Therefore, it is important to pretreat the instruments with enzymatic solution as soon as feasibly possible, preferably prior to transport from the operating room to the central processing area. Remember, enzymatic solution is not a disinfectant; it is just a way to help break down dried blood or debris.

CLEANING/DECONTAMINATION PROCESSES

Manual Cleaning

Some instruments are manually cleaned, based upon the manufacturer's instructions for use (also called *IFU*), which are the manufacturer's recommendations. Some instruments that are manually cleaned include:

- Laparoscopes
- Cords
- Camera heads
- Delicate instruments
- Power saws or drills

Detergents that are used on any instrument or equipment should have the following characteristics:

- Neutral pH of 7
- Low foam
- Rinse easily
- Nonabrasive
- Nontoxic
- Biodegradable
- Cost-effective

Ultrasonic Cleaning

Some instruments that cannot withstand mechanical cleaning, need to be placed in an ultrasonic cleaner. The ultrasonic cleaner works by cavitation, which is a process that creates small bubbles that implode. This creates a suction-like action that pulls the debris from the instrument surface. An ultrasonic detergent is added to the water to aid in the cleaning process. Upon removal from the ultrasonic cleaner, the instruments must be rinsed with pure water. It is recommended that all laparoscopic instruments receive ultrasonic cleaning.

Final Rinse of All Instruments

All instruments that were manually, ultrasonically, or mechanically cleaned must go through a final rinse with pure water to remove any residuals that could stain the instruments or affect sterilization. Pure water can be:

- Reverse-osmosis water
- Deionized water
- Distilled water

Mechanical Cleaning

The instruments, depending upon the manufacturer's instructions for use, are placed in a washer/disinfector or a washer/sterilizer, whereby they are treated with an enzymatic cleaner and a detergent during an automated process that uses hot water (approximately 150°F to 170°F or 65°C to 77°C).

Washer-Decontamination Cycles

Each washer/disinfector or washer/sterilizer has different yet similar cycles to clean and decontaminate the instrumentation and equipment. Some such cycles are:

- Cool-water rinse to remove any debris
- Enzymatic rinse
- Detergent wash
- Ultrasonic clean
- Hot-water rinse
- Deionized-water final rinse
- Lubrication rinse
- Dry cycle
- Sterilization (only on washer/sterilizer units)

Essential Facts

Question: A tray of specialty instruments was used for a surgery and the surgeon would like you to wash the instruments between the cases in the operating room. What should you do?

Answer: These instruments need to go to the central processing area of the hospital where they are treated with the enzymatic solution, detergent, and all other necessary steps prior to sterilization. Washing instruments between surgeries in the operating room is discouraged and should be done only in emergency situations.

PREPARATION AND PACKAGING

After the instruments and equipment are cleaned and decontaminated, it is time to prepare and package them properly for the sterilization process. Each instrument or piece of equipment should be inspected for:

- Cleanliness
- Proper alignment
- Corrosion, cracks, pitting, and rust
- Sharpness
- Loose screws
- Wear and tear
- Missing pieces
- Overall functionality

This will ensure that the instrument tray or piece of equipment opened on the sterile field will be optimum for use. It is also important to make sure that the instrument or piece of equipment is completely dry before packaging. Any residual moisture can create damage, such as rust, pitting, or compromise the sterility of the item.

Essential Facts

After surgical scissors have been in use for a while, the sharp cutting edge will become dull and under magnification will look rounded off and may have formed pits. Because this is not visible with the naked eye, in central processing, it is important to test each scissor by cutting the appropriate testing material for the specific scissor. The testing material is designed to especially test even the most delicate scissors. The cutting action should be smooth as the scissor closes and should not grind, jump, feel loose, or feel too tight. The scissors should not pinch or grate the testing material. If the scissors are working well, they will produce a nice and straight cut.

Preparation

Instruments should be packaged so that the sterilant comes in contact with *all* exposed surfaces. Packaging requirements include:

- The container must be large enough so that instruments are contained in a single layer.
- The instruments should be placed on their sides to facilitate drying (steam sterilization).

- Hinges should be open. An instrument stringer should be used to ensure ring-handled instruments are kept in the open position.
- Stopcocks should be in the open position, so that all surfaces are completely exposed to the sterilant.
- Perforated tip protectors should be placed on delicate or sharp instruments.
- Heavy instruments should be placed at the bottom of the tray, unless indicated otherwise by the manufacturer's IFU.

Items that should *not* be used when packaging instruments for sterilization include:

- Rubber bands around instruments
- Paper/plastic peel-packages used to segregate instruments within the tray
- Stylets in lumen items, unless manufacturer's IFU specifically recommends leaving it in

Specialty Equipment

Power equipment (e.g., drills, saws) should be sterilized according to the manufacturer's IFU and be lubricated and tested before sterilization. This will increase the life expectancy of the power equipment.

Scopes and cords should be cleaned according to the manufacturer's IFU and checked for visibility and functionality before sterilization.

Ophthalmic instruments require specific care due to toxic anterior segment syndrome (TASS). This is a contaminant that is introduced to the eye, due to the inadequate cleaning, rinsing, and sterilization process of eye surgery instruments. Often, single-use items, especially with lumens, are used to reduce the risk.

Packaging

Packaging materials can be:

- Single-use nonwoven material
- Multiuse woven textile (not as common)

Basic guidelines for packaging of instruments and equipment are often dependent upon the type of sterilization process used. Some general guidelines are:

- Trays should not weigh over 25 pounds.
- Trays should include a proper indicator for the sterilization modality.
- Trays should be labeled with product identification, lot number, and process date.

Indicators

Indicators are types of monitoring devices that offer evidence that the sterilization process has occurred.

There are three different types of indicators used during the sterilization process:

- Chemical: Validates one or more parameters typically with a color change
- Biological: Validates sterilization by achieving microbial kill
- Mechanical: Sterilizer sensor prints out and alarms

Type 5 integrators are the most widely used as they measure time, temperature, and pressure.

Chemical indicators are placed inside and outside of a package prior to sterilization. The chemical indicator undergoes a visual color change if a package was exposed to the proper physical conditions of sterilization (temperature, pressure, and time). Note that chemical indicators do not guarantee sterility.

Biological indicators are used in every load. This requires placing a prepackaged, self-contained vial of a bacterial spore in an appropriate test/challenge pack—*Bacillus stearothermophilus* for steam sterilizers or *Bacillus subtilis var. niger* for ethylene oxide (EtO) sterilizers—in the sterilizer for a cycle to see whether the cycle kills all the spores. If it does, then the sterilizer is working properly. The results from the biological indicator must be *negative* and the load should not be released and/or utilized until a negative result is confirmed.

Mechanical indicators, Bowie–Dick tests, are used daily to monitor the function of the steam sterilizers. Sterilizer program parameters, specifically Bowie–Dick tests, are used to validate the efficacy of the prevac cycle of these sterilizers. This test consists of a series of air removal and steam penetration barriers with a chemical indicator in the center of each pack. The pack is placed directly into an empty steam sterilizer to see whether the steam displaces the air through the barrier material within the pack. A uniform change in color from yellow to blue/purple on the indicator sheet indicates that all the air was displaced and the appropriate vacuum was achieved for optimal steam penetration.

Validation of the sterilization cycle should include chemical and biological indicators, and mechanical monitoring of the sterilizer.

STERILIZATION

Within an organization, sterilization cycles include different parameters for different types of sterilization. Common types of sterilization are:

- Steam
- Gravity displacement
- Chemical
- Ethylene oxide

To determine the type of sterilization necessary for instruments or devices, it is important to look at the manufacturer's instructions for use for compatibility and specific parameters. Some instruments and equipment that are commonly steam sterilized are:

- Stainless steel or laparoscopic instrument trays
- Some scopes
- Drills, saws, and other power equipment

Some instruments and equipment that are commonly chemically sterilized are:

- Laparoscopes
- Camera heads
- Flexible scopes
- Batteries for power equipment

Parameters for the different types of sterilization are shown in Tables 8.1 through 8.5. Parameters for hydrogen peroxide plasma sterilization are set by the sterilizer manufacturer. They should fall within the ranges shown in Table 8.4.

Table 8.1

Gravity-Displacement Steam Sterilization Parameters

Item Type	Exposure Time at 250°F or 121°C	Exposure Time at 270°F or 132°C	Exposure Time at 275°F or 135°C	Dry Time
Wrapped instrument tray	30 min	15 min	10 min	15–30 min 30 min
Textile pack	30 min	25 min	10 min	15 min 30 min
Unwrapped instruments		3 min	3 min	0–1 min
Unwrapped porous item or lumen/cannula item		10 min	10 min	0–1 min

Table 8.2
Parameters for Dynamic Air-Removal Steam Sterilization

Item Type	Exposure Time at 270°F or 132°C	Exposure Time at 275°F or 135°C	Dry Time
Wrapped instrument tray	4 min	3 min	20–30 min 16 min
Textile pack	4 min	3 min	5–20 min 3 min
Unwrapped instruments	3 min	3 min	None
Unwrapped porous item or lumen/cannula item	4 min	3 min	None

Table 8.3
Parameters for Ethylene Oxide Chemical Sterilization

Humidity	Temperature	Exposure Time	Aeration Time
50%–75%	85°F–145°F 30°C–63°C	2 hr	8 hr at 140°F/60°C 12 hr at 122°F/50°C

Table 8.4
Parameters for Vaporized Hydrogen Peroxide Sterilization

Temperature	Time
104°F–131°F 40°C–55°C	28–75 min

Table 8.5
Parameters for Peracetic Acid Sterilization

Temperature	Time
122°F–131°F 50°C–55°C	12 min

Exhibit 8.1

Handling of Flexible Endoscopes

A northeastern Illinois hospital had a cluster of carbapenem-resistant Enterobacteriaceae [CRE] outbreaks in 2013, the Centers for Disease Control and Prevention launched an investigation and traced it back to a duodenoscope used during an endoscopic retrograde cholangiopancreatography (ECRP). This hospital moved from using high-level disinfection, using an automated endoscope reprocessors (AERs), to using EtO gas sterilization when duodenoscopes were used on patients with known CRE infection. Additional CRE outbreaks followed during 2015 in the United States and were also traced to duodenoscopes that were not adequately reprocessed. Therefore, some hospitals are now looking toward using disposable duodenoscopes or at minimum, disposable distal covers to make it easier to clean. The following process should be used when handling any flexible endoscope:

- It is imperative to preclean flexible endoscopes and accessories at the point of use or as soon as possible.
- Process flexible endoscopes and accessories as soon as transported.
- Leak testing should be performed right before manual cleaning and before the endoscope is placed into cleaning solutions.
- All accessible channels and the distal end of the endoscope should be cleaned with an appropriate-sized cleaning brush.
- Endoscope valves should be manually actuated during cleaning.
- Channels of the endoscope should be flushed with cleaning solution.
- Perform manual cleaning verification process after manual cleaning to test for remaining residual organic debris (Petersen et al., 2017).
- AER or EtO specifically for duodenoscopes should be used according to manufacturer's IFU.
- Integrity of flexible endoscope should be visually inspected and hung in a drying cabinet with all valves open, and removable parts should be detached if AER is used for high-level disinfection.
- If duodenoscope is EtO gas sterilized, it should be stored in a manner that minimizes contamination and protects the scope from damage (Rahman et al., 2019).

Immediate-Use Steam Sterilization

Unwrapped sterilization takes place when an item is dropped during surgery or when a tray of instruments or equipment needs to be processed right away. This is considered *immediate-use steam sterilization (IUSS)* and is discouraged except in emergency situations. It was formerly called *flash sterilization*.

Advantages and Disadvantages of Sterilization Types

Both steam and chemical sterilization have many advantages and disadvantages.

Common advantages of steam sterilization are:

- Nontoxic
- Cost-effective
- Penetrates packaging and lumens/cannulas
- Large capacity sterilizers are available

Common disadvantages of steam sterilization are:

- Damages heat-sensitive items
- Can lead to moisture in packages
- Has the potential to burn staff

Common advantages of EtO chemical sterilization are:

- Compatible with most materials
- Penetrates packaging and lumen/cannulas
- Simple to operate and monitor

Common disadvantages of EtO chemical sterilization are:

- Requires aeration time to remove EtO residue
- Toxic, uses a carcinogen, and flammable
- Long sterilization process
- Burdensome regulatory monitoring required

Common advantages of vaporized hydrogen peroxide sterilization are:

- Environmentally safe
- Nontoxic, no venting required
- Short cycle time

Common disadvantages of vaporized hydrogen peroxide sterilization are:

- Cannot process textiles, liquids, or anything containing absorbable items
- Cannot process some long lumens
- Requires special packaging
- Small capacity

Common advantages of peracetic acid sterilization are:

- Quick turnaround time
- Less damaging to instruments
- Easy to use

Common disadvantages of peracetic acid sterilization are:

- Can only be used with instruments that can be immersed
- Potential for eye and skin damage
- May be materials compatibility concerns for lead, brass, copper, and zinc
- Immediate use only, cannot be stored sterile

STERILE STORAGE

After instruments and equipment are sterilized, it is important to store them in the proper place.

The temperature of the storage area should be approximately 75°F (24°C) and the humidity should not exceed 70%.

Other guidelines include:

- Use a maintenance cover (dust cover) on items that are not commonly used to insure package integrity.
- Keep items in closed or covered cabinets.
- Shelves, if racks, should be clean and dry with plastic shelf liners used to protect packages from becoming perforated.
- Supplies should be rotated.
- Touch supplies with clean hands.

Stringent guidelines are followed and a great deal of care is involved in the processing of sterile instruments and equipment used during the surgical procedure. Properly processing instruments and equipment is an important measure to prevent surgical-site infections and promote patient safety. It is important to be able to distinguish between sterile and nonsterile items through visibly identifying chemical indicators in order to prevent nonsterile items from entering a sterile field.

References

Petersen, B. T., Cohen, J., Hambrick, R. D., Buttar, N., Greenwald, D. A., Buscaglia, J. M., ... & Eisen, G. (2017). Multisociety guideline on reprocessing flexible GI endoscopes: 2016 update. *Gastrointestinal endoscopy, 85*(2), 282–294.

Rahman, M. R., Perisetti, A., Coman, R., Bansal, P., Chhabra, R., & Goyal, H. (2019). Duodenoscope-associated infections: update on an emerging problem. *Digestive diseases and sciences, 64*(6), 1409–1418.

9

Surgical Supplies

Various surgical supplies are needed for each surgical procedure. It is the responsibility of the scrub nurse/certified surgical technologist (CST) and the circulating nurse to have everything ready that may be needed for the procedure. There are also many surgical supplies that should be available at all times to keep the patient safe.

During this part of your orientation, you will learn about:

- Different types of surgical supplies
- General guidelines for supplies
- Handling of implants and tissue
- Surgical inventory systems

SPONGES

Sponges are a mainstay in the operating room used to absorb blood and body fluids, create a clear field for the surgeon to work, and apply pressure to control bleeding. They are sterile and made of highly absorbent gauze material. They come in multiple sizes and shapes to be used in many different areas of the body. These sponges are x-ray detectable, meaning that blue threads made of polypropylene, polyester, and barium sulfate are woven into the sponge and are visible upon x-ray. This is useful if a sponge is inadvertently left in a patient in that it will be detected upon x-ray examination. Table 9.1 lists common types of sponges and their uses.

Table 9.1

Common Sponges and Their Usage

Name of Sponge	Shape	Common Usage
4 × 4	Square that is 4 inches by 4 inches	Minor surgery
Laparotomy pad ("lap pad")	Rectangular-shaped gauze with a band and ring attached to the corner	Abdominal surgery
Laminectomy pad ("lami pad")	Smaller version of the lap pad	Spinal surgery Pediatric surgery
Peanut "kittner"	Tightly woven gauze about 5 mm in diameter	Blunt dissection Head and neck surgery
Round balls	Cotton-filled gauze ball about 20 mm in diameter	Pelvic surgery
Tonsil rod	Cylindrical-shaped sponge with string	Tonsil surgery
Tonsil ball	Ball-shaped sponge with string	Tonsil surgery
Cottonoid ("cotton pattie")	Many different-sized, thin cotton pads that are attached to a string	Neurosurgery Nasal surgery

SHARPS

Sharp surgical supplies include knife blades and sutures.

Knife Blades

Knife blades come in many different shapes and sizes. They are commonly made of carbon steel and must be very sharp.

Commonly used knife blades are:

- 20 blade (common for skin incision)
- 10 blade (Figure 9.1)
- 15 blade (Figure 9.1)
- 11 blade (Figure 9.1)
- 12 blade
- Beaver blade (common for eyes, ears)

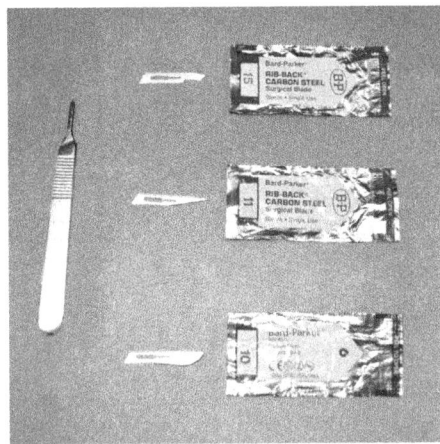

Figure 9.1 Knife handle (*left*), 15 blade (*top*), 11 blade (*middle*), and 10 blade (*bottom*).

- Lancet blade
- Sickle blade

Sutures and Needles

Sutures are used to anastomose or close tissue. They come in many different styles, and their usage in specific procedures is dependent on the following:

- Anatomic site
- Type of tissue
- Surgeon's preference
- Required suture characteristics

Suture Characteristics

- Absorbent natural or synthetic dissolve over time commonly used on soft tissue such as adipose tissue, subcutaneous tissue, and intestinal tissue
- Nonabsorbent natural or synthetic do not dissolve commonly used on cardiovascular tissue, neurological tissue, and the skin

Some absorbent natural sutures:

- Collagen
- Plain surgical gut
- Fast-absorbing surgical gut
- Chronic surgical gut

Some absorbent synthetic sutures are:

- Polyglactin 910 (Vicryl)
- Polycaprolate (Dexon II)
- Poliglecaprone 25 (Monocryl)

Some nonabsorbent natural sutures:

- Surgical silk
- Surgical cotton
- Surgical steel

Some nonabsorbent synthetic sutures:

- Nylon
- Polyester fiber (Mersilene/Surgidac uncoated and Ethibond/Ti-cron coated)
- Polypropylene (Prolene)

Sutures can also be:

- Monofilament (e.g., Prolene)
- Multifilament (e.g., silk)

Each suture is usually attached to a needle (Figure 9.2). The needles come in different:

- Tips
- Body types
- Swag types
- Sizes

If the suture is not attached to a needle it is called a *free tie*. A free tie may come in a package on a reel (Figure 9.3) or just in a package. Free ties are used in conjunction with clamps to tie off small vessels.

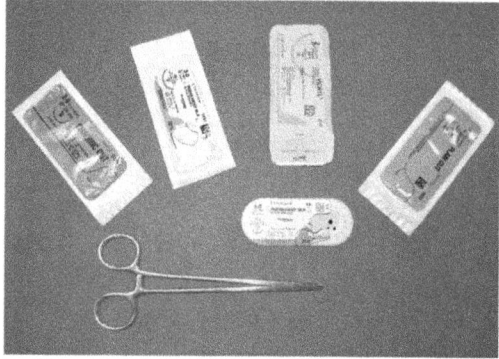

Figure 9.2 Suture with needle.

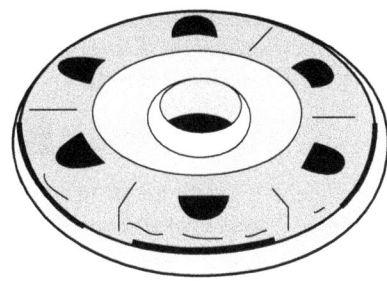

Figure 9.3 Suture reel.

Some newer techniques incorporate the use of a closure device that is suture material with barbs that can be bidirectional and unidirectional, as well as knotless sutures. The suture has anchors incorporated into the suture material to create consistent tension and enhance strength. These closure devices can save time and help create a strong suture line.

Essential Facts

At first, use of sutures and needles is usually confusing in the operating room. After a while, it becomes easier to understand and remember what type of suture is used on specific types of tissue. One easy thing to remember is that absorbent sutures are not usually used on blood vessels because when they dissolve, it could cause the suture line to fail.

Syringes and Needles

Syringes come in all shapes and sizes; the choice of syringe is dependent upon how much fluid is being drawn up for the patient. Some common syringe sizes are:

- 1 mL or tuberculin
- 3 mL
- 5 mL
- 10 mL
- 20 mL
- 60 mL

Needles that can be attached to the syringes can either be:

- An active or passive needle-based safety device (recommended)
- A regular plain needle with no safety device

The diameter of each needle is measured as its gauge (G). The higher the number (e.g., 22 G) the smaller the diameter of the needle. This is opposite to the gauging of French catheter sizes.

Essential Facts

Question: The surgeon is asking for an 18-G needle and a 24-G needle. Which one will have a smaller diameter?
Answer: The 24-G needle has a smaller diameter.

Suction Tubing

Suction tubing should be available in the operating room at all times. It is used on the sterile field to remove fluid or blood. It is also used by the anesthesia provider to suction the airway. Having a supply of suction tubing is very important, especially in an emergency. It is also recommended to have suction set up and ready to go whenever a patient comes into the operating room.

Sterile Covers

There are many different types of sterile covers, which are placed over items that are introduced to the sterile field. Some such items include:

- Probe cover
- Microscope cover
- Camera cover
- Light handle cover

Catheters

Catheters come in many different sizes and can be used for many different purposes, such as to drain urine, fluid, or blood from a patient. Some such catheters include:

- Urinary catheters
- Red rubber catheters ("straight catheters")
- Malecot catheters
- Pigtail catheters
- Coude catheters

It is important to remember that the sizing of the catheters is represented in French (F) gauge. The larger the number (e.g., 24 F) the larger the diameter of the catheter. This is the opposite of needle measurements, and sometimes can confuse new operating room nurses.

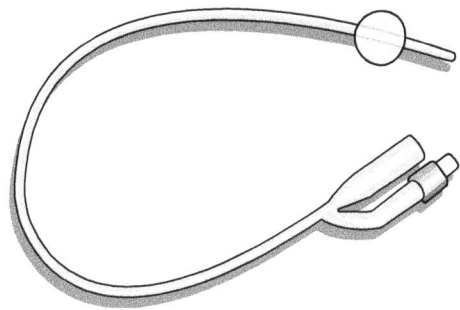

Figure 9.4 Urinary catheter hub and balloon tip.

Another important aspect of catheters is the balloon sometimes found on the tip of the catheter (Figure 9.4). The purpose of this balloon is usually to secure the catheter in the cavity or to apply pressure to the wall of the cavity. Each balloon has a maximum capacity of fluid (sterile water) or air that can go into it. This amount will be on the hub of the fluid port and also on the packaging description.

Essential Facts

It is important to remember to use sterile water and not sterile saline in balloon catheters because saline in the balloon can corrode the rubber catheter. Also, even though the balloon holds a specific amount of fluid, additional fluid will need to be inserted to fill the channel of the catheter. Example: A 5-mL balloon will come with a 10-mL syringe of sterile water; 5 mL ends up in the balloon and 5 mL fills the channel leading up to the balloon.

Drains

Drains are used to:

- Prevent a fluid accumulation such as blood or serum
- Prevent air accumulation within the body cavity, also called *dead space*

Drains can be:

- Open, meaning not connected to anything (e.g., Penrose)
- Closed, meaning connected to a collection device (e.g., Jackson-Pratt)

The collection device can be:

- Passive, just collecting fluid (e.g., T tube)
- Active, whereby it is suctioning out fluid (e.g., Hemovac)

Other Accessories

There are many other sterile supplies that are brought into the operating room or may even be a main staple in the room. Some such items include:

- Procedural trays
- Specimen containers
- Vessel loops
- Anti-fog devices
- Cautery tip cleaners
- Waterproof skin markers
- Applicator sticks
- Safety pins

GENERAL GUIDELINES FOR STERILE SUPPLIES

Some general guidelines should be followed when sterile supplies are used. These guidelines include:

- Keep supplies in a closed cabinet in the operating room.
- Discard any supplies left in the room that were not utilized if a patient was in the operating room.
- Have the material safety data sheets and instructions for use on file and available for review.

Essential Facts

Question: Why is it important to anticipate and gather surgical supplies before the patient arrives in the operating room?
Answer: Once the patient arrives in the operating room, you will be giving the patient and the surgical team your undivided attention. Also, leaving the room will increase traffic and movement, which can increase shedding of microbes (see Chapter 6).

IMPLANTS

The U.S. Food and Drug Administration (FDA) states that any permanently implantable device must be documented on an implant log for tracking purposes. Unique device identifiers (UDIs) are required by the FDA to be on the label and packaging of implants so that they can be placed into the FDA's Global UDI Database.

Implants include:

- Medical devices
- Tissue
- Bone
- Synthetic or biological grafts

Documentation should include:

- Location of implant
- Name of manufacturer
- Lot and/or serial number
- Type and/or size of implant
- Expiration date, if applicable

Tissue banks are treated a bit differently and fall under the auspices of the American Association of Tissue Banks.

Tissues that may be kept in a bank can include:

- Corneal tissue
- Stem cells
- Bone

The AATB requires:

- Copies of the AATB accreditation of outside vendors from which the tissue is obtained
- Copies of the FDA registration
- Listings of all tissue products ordered, stored, and used

Quality control and tracking of both implants and tissue can be automated or manual; either way, it is important to accurately document them in order to be able to retrieve correct information in the event of a recall.

SURGICAL INVENTORY SYSTEMS

Automating supplies helps to control the inventory of surgical supplies and capture valuable usage information for charging patient accounts and reordering inventory.

Surgical inventory systems can:

- Reduce inventory on hand
- Produce monthly reports
- Reduce workflow interruptions
- Charge patient accounts immediately upon usage
- Reduce loss of charges

These types of systems are a proactive approach to efficiently manage supplies. It is important for the scrub nurse/CST, RN first assistant, and circulating nurse to be able to navigate the surgical inventory system. Most systems provide online training and are not difficult to navigate.

III

Surgical Basics

10

Basic Surgical Procedures

There are many different types of surgical procedures. It is important to understand basic anatomy and physiology, patient risk factors, and the different surgical interventions that are available to the patient. Over the past few decades, surgery has evolved to become minimally invasive and more technologically driven. The RN, certified surgical technologist, and first assistant should understand basic surgical procedures and be able to adapt their understanding of these basic procedures to different patient populations.

During this part of your orientation, you will learn about:

- The basic categories of surgical procedures
- Identifying patient position, draping, and supplies
- General age-appropriate considerations

Understanding surgical procedures takes a great deal of time and knowledge. At the beginning, it is important to understand basic categories and be able to identify and anticipate specific patient needs.

OTOLARYNGOLOGY, HEAD, AND NECK PROCEDURES

Some common otolaryngology, head, and neck procedures include:

- Tonsillectomy
- Nasal reconstruction
- Facial reconstruction

- Stapedectomy (middle ear procedure)
- Thyroidectomy and parathyroidectomy
- Neck dissection

Common positions for these types of procedures are:

- Supine
- Semi-Fowler's, also known as *beach chair*

Common drapes for these types of procedures are:

- Head drape
- U drape
- Body sheet

A head drape (Figure 10.1) helps keep the patient's hair out of the sterile field. Hair is considered unsanitary and should be contained in a disposable hair cover and sterile drapes. A head drape can be made with:

- Two towels
- A towel and a ¾ sheet
- A non-perforating plastic towel clip used to hold the drape closed

Supplies will vary depending upon the procedure and the surgeon's preference, but common supplies include:

- Electrocautery with needle tip
- Peanuts to bluntly dissect (head and neck procedures)
- Absorbent sutures
- Vessel loops
- Specialty instrument trays

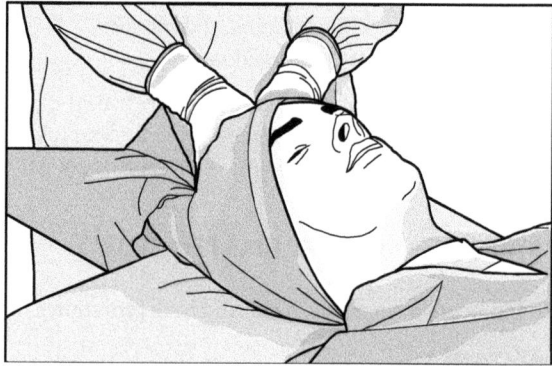

Figure 10.1 Head drape.

- Implants (facial reconstruction procedures)
- Tonsil sponges
- Cottonoids (nasal procedures)

OPHTHALMIC PROCEDURES

Some common ophthalmic procedures include:

- Cataract surgery
- Dacrocystorhinostomy (creation of new tear duct into the nasal cavity)
- Excision of chalazion (eyelid cyst)
- Blepharoplasty (eyelid surgery)
- Enucleation (removal of an eyeball)
- Exenteration (removal of orbit)
- Keratoplasty (removal/replacement of the cornea)

Common positions for these types of procedures are:

- Supine
- Semi-Fowler's, also known as *beach chair*

Many times, the patient's head needs to be stabilized by using a strap or holder; padded wrist straps are also used to hold the patient in position. Some operating room beds have a narrow headpiece that allows the surgeon to move closer to the operative eye.

Common drapes for these types of procedures are:

- Head drape
- U drape
- Body sheet
- Plastic eye drape to repel fluid
- Cardboard bridge

The cardboard bridge will be placed on the patient's chin to prop the drape up so that it does not lay on the patient's nose or mouth. This will afford the patient more comfort during the procedure.

Supplies will vary depending upon the procedure and the surgeon's preference, but common supplies include:

- Microscope drape
- Weck-Cel
- Implants
- Disposable eye knives and needles
- Balanced salt irrigating solution (BSS)

> **Essential Facts**
>
> BSS is an isotonic solution used in irrigating tissues of the eyes. It is used as both an extraocular (outside) and intraocular (inside) irrigation solution of the eye. This helps keep the eye moist. Normally, people blink 2 to 50 times a minute to keep the eye moist and clean. Because the eye is held open during ophthalmic procedures and a microscope light is shining directly on the eye, it is important to provide moisture by irrigating the eye with BSS.

Specialty equipment used depends upon the type of ophthalmic procedure. The perioperative staff must be competent in setting up and working with each specific machine.

Specialty equipment includes:

- Phacoemulsification machine (cataract procedures)
- Posterior vitrectomy machine (vitrectomy procedures)
- Cryotherapy machine (retinal procedures)
- Lasers (postcataract procedures, corneal procedures, and vitrectomy procedures)

CARDIAC, THORACIC, AND VASCULAR PROCEDURES

Some common cardiac, thoracic, and vascular procedures include:

- Bronchoscopy (visualization of trachea, bronchi, and lungs)
- Thoracotomy (incision into the thorax, possibly for a biopsy)
- Pneumonectomy (removal of a lung)
- Coronary artery bypass graft (open heart surgery to improve blood flow)
- Mitral valve replacement (replacement of a heart valve)
- Femoral–popliteal bypass (restoring blood flow to the leg by using a graft to bypass the occluded area)

Common positions for these types of procedures are:

- Supine
- Lateral with operative side up
- Semilateral with operative side up

Common drapes for these types of procedures are:

- Towels
- Fenestrated drape
- Body drape

Supplies will vary depending upon the procedure and the surgeon's preference, but common supplies include:

- Lap pads
- Vessel loops
- Round balls on sponge sticks
- Electrocautery
- Staple devices
- Fiberoptic scopes
- Sutures with pledgets
- Chest tube and drainage system

A chest tube and chest drainage system is utilized whenever the chest cavity is opened. This will restore the negative pressure and prevent the lungs from collapsing. The chest tube is placed in the patient at the end of the surgical procedure and hooked up to the chest drainage system when the chest is closed (Figure 10.2).

Specialty equipment needed depends upon the type of procedure but may include:

- Cardiac bypass machine
- Additional monitoring equipment
- Doppler ultrasound

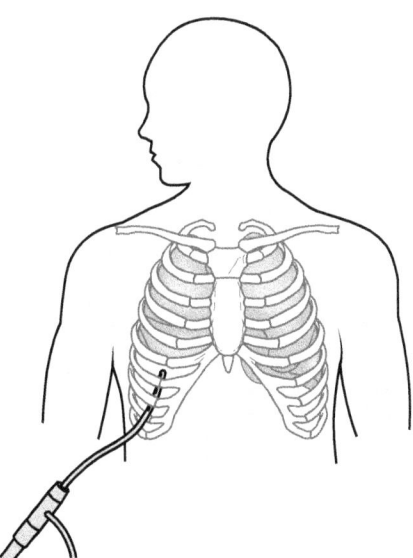

Figure 10.2 Chest tube device and placement.

> **Essential Facts**
>
> A Doppler ultrasound uses sound waves to determine how well blood flows through a blood vessel. The surgeon can determine a blockage or reduced blood flow while in the operating room and can reevaluate the vessel, if necessary. Doppler equipment can be sterile for use intraoperatively or be used unsterile at the end of the surgical procedure to confirm blood flow.

GENERAL AND ABDOMINAL PROCEDURES

Some common general and abdominal procedures include:

- Mastectomy (removal of breast)
- Herniorraphy (repair of hernia)
- Cholecystectomy (removal of gallbladder)
- Colon resection (removal of a portion of intestines)
- Appendectomy (removal of appendix)
- Abdominal aortic aneurysm resection (removal of a weakened wall of the aorta with placement of a graft)

Common positions for these types of procedures are:

- Supine
- Lithotomy

Common drapes for these types of procedures are:

- Towels
- Fenestrated drape
- Body drape

Supplies will vary depending upon the procedure and the surgeon's preference, but common supplies include:

- Electrocautery
- Lap pads
- Round balls on sponge sticks
- Energy devices
- Implantable grafts, mesh
- Stapling devices for anastomosis

Laparoscopic Procedures

Due to advances in surgical technique, many abdominal procedures are now performed laparoscopically. This allows patients to have a much shorter recovery time and less pain postoperatively. Some additional supplies necessary for laparoscopic procedures are:

- Scopes and cameras
- Veress needle for insufflation
- Trocars

Scopes come in many different diameter sizes (e.g., 2, 5, 10 mm) and have different optical angle views (e.g., 0°, 30°, 45°, 70°). These optical angle views are dependent upon what field of view the surgeon would like for the procedure. Scopes can also come in extended lengths (e.g., 31, 42, 57 cm) for deeper cavities.

Trocars provide access to the abdominal cavity through a very small incision. In order to be able to place trocars in the abdominal cavity, it is first important to insufflate the abdomen with carbon dioxide gas. The veress needle is small and blunt so it can go in gently to safely access the intraabdominal cavity. Once the abdomen is sufficiently insufflated, then the trocars can be introduced. Sometimes, trocars are placed without insufflation, but care must be taken to avoid puncturing any abdominal structures (e.g., colon, aorta).

Insufflation is the instilling of (preferably warm) carbon dioxide gas into the abdominal cavity to help visualize anatomy and create a space to perform surgery. This process is called *pneumoperitoneum*. Carbon dioxide gas is used because it is

- Noncombustible
- Easily absorbed
- Inexpensive

Caution must be taken when controlling the insufflator, and monitoring of the following is imperative for patient safety:

- Flow rate (usually about 15 to 20 L/min)
- Total volume (varies with length of procedure)
- Intraabdominal pressure (approximately 15 mmHg)

Trocars allow the surgeon to make a small incision and then pass long instruments through the portal to perform surgery. There are many different types of trocars. Trocars can be

- Sharp
- Blunt or bladeless
- Dilating

Trocars also come in many different sizes, ranging from 5 to 12 mm, depending upon what scope or instrumentation will be passed through.

The components of the trocar are

- Sheath or sleeve
- Obturator

Many trocars are now resposable, whereby part of the trocar is disposed of and part of the trocar is reusable. Reducer caps are also available and designed to snap onto the open end of a trocar sleeve and reduce the opening to a small size. This will prevent gas from escaping from the abdominal cavity and losing distention, meaning that the carbon dioxide gas escapes through the trocar, therefore compromising the visualization of the abdominal structures.

Essential Facts

Question: A new nurse has just received an assignment to prepare an operating room for a colon resection on a 58-year-old patient with a history of multiple abdominal procedures. What are some important considerations?

Answer: The new nurse would first need to find out whether the surgery will be performed laparoscopically or open. Due to the history of multiple abdominal procedures, the patient may have adhesions. Therefore, it would be prudent for the nurse to have the supplies and equipment for an open procedure available, which would include electrocautery, lap pads, the surgeon's preferred energy devices, staples, trocars, scopes, and cameras.

GYNECOLOGICAL AND GENITOURINARY PROCEDURES

Some common gynecological and genitourinary procedures include:

- Hysterectomy (removal of the uterus)
- Salpingo-oophorectomy (removal of the fallopian tube and ovary)
- Dilatation and curettage (dilating of the uterine cervix and scraping of the endometrial lining of the uterus)
- Prostatectomy (removal of the prostate)
- Transurethral resection of prostate or bladder tumor (removal of the prostate or bladder tumor through the urethra)

Common positions for these types of procedures are:

- Supine
- Lithotomy

Common drapes for these types of procedures are:

- Towels
- Fenestrated drape
- Body drape

Supplies will vary depending upon the procedure and the surgeon's preference, but common supplies include:

- Electrocautery
- Lap pads

- Round balls on sponge sticks
- Energy devices

ROBOTIC SURGERY

As mentioned in the previous section, many surgical procedures are commonly performed laparoscopically. Some surgeons are also utilizing robot technology for these procedures. Robotic surgery utilizes robotic devices that assist the surgeon by holding and maneuvering laparoscopic instrumentation. In some cases, robotic surgery can result in a smaller incision and provide more precision and enhanced dexterity for the surgeon.

Some common laparoscopic surgeries that can be done robotically are:

- Hysterectomy (removal of the uterus)
- Prostatectomy (removal of the prostate)
- Nephrectomy (removal of the kidney)

ORTHOPEDIC PROCEDURES

Some common orthopedic procedures include:

- Hip or knee replacement
- Laminectomy (removal of a disc from the cervical, thoracic, or lumbar spine)
- External fixator (applying a surgical device externally to hold a fracture in place while it heals)
- Arthroscopy (visualize a joint with a scope)
- Open reduction internal fixation (reduce a fracture and stabilize it with screws, pins, and/or plates)

Common positions for these types of procedures are:

- Supine
- Semi-Fowler's
- Fracture table with traction

For certain types of fractures, a specialized fracture table is used that enables the surgeon to put the extremity under traction during the surgery to align the fracture. This is commonly done under continuous x-ray visualization, also known as *fluoroscopy*.

Common drapes for these types of procedures are:

- Towels
- Fenestrated drape
- Impervious drapes due to fluid loss (e.g., body fluid, irrigation)
- Body drape

Supplies will vary depending upon the procedure and the surgeon's preference, but common supplies include:

- Electrocautery
- Lap pads
- Implants

NEUROSURGERY PROCEDURES

Some common neurosurgery procedures include:

- Craniotomy (incision into the cranium to perform surgery on the brain)
- Cranioplasty (repair of a skull defect, possibly due to trauma, malformation, or prior surgical procedure)
- Spinal fusion (the fusing together of two or more vertebrae)

Common positions for these types of procedures are:

- Supine
- Prone
- Fowler's

Common drapes for these types of procedures are:

- Towels
- Fenestrated drape
- Impervious drapes due to fluid loss (e.g., body fluid, irrigation)
- Body drape

Supplies will vary depending upon the procedure and the surgeon's preference, but common supplies include:

- Electrocautery
- Lami pads
- Cottonoids

GENERAL AGE-APPROPRIATE CONSIDERATIONS

Each patient should be treated individually based on:

- Age
- Mental status
- Cognitive development
- Cultural beliefs
- Personal limitations

Some general considerations for neonates, infants, and pediatric patients include:

- Maintaining normothermia
- Using small drapes and supplies due to small surface area
- Using developmentally appropriate words when speaking with a child

Some general considerations for elderly patients include

- Maintaining normothermia
- Assessing and monitoring fragile skin integrity
- Assessing range of motion and positioning accordingly
- Considering osteoporosis and potential for fractures

Some general consideration for bariatric patients (body mass index that is equal to or greater than 30) include:

- Using specialty equipment (e.g., large stretcher, large operating room bed, oversized gowns, oversized blood pressure cuff)
- Using extra-long instrumentation
- Using an air-assisted transfer device or a power lifter device
- Securing enough personnel to assist

Essential Facts

Question: The nurse is discussing a right inguinal hernia repair with a 6-year-old patient. Which explanation would be appropriate?
Explanation 1: "We are going to put you under anesthesia and surgically repair your right inguinal hernia. Then you will arrive in the postanesthesia care unit, where you will emerge from the anesthetic."
Explanation 2: "We are going to have you take a little nap, while we fix your tummy. When you wake up, you will be with your family in the 'wake-up room.' We will take great care of you."
Answer: Explanation 2 is age appropriate for a 6-year-old child.

LASER PROCEDURES

Lasers are used in many different types of surgical specialties, including:

- Ophthalmology
- Otolaryngology
- Gynecology
- Urology

The word *laser* is an acronym for "light amplification by stimulated emission of radiation." The laser produces light when energy is added to a medium. This causes the release of energy in the form of a narrow beam of high-energy light that has a thermal effect on tissue to cut, coagulate, or vaporize.

Laser energy can be:

- Infrared
- Ultraviolet
- Visible

The light can have different interactions with tissue; it can:

- Reflect
- Scatter
- Transmit
- Absorb

Therefore, lasers must be used with caution and can be dangerous, possibly causing the following:

- Eye injury to the cornea and retina
- Skin burns
- Surgical smoke hazards
- Fire hazards

Hospitals should have a laser safety program, interdisciplinary laser committee, and an appointed a laser safety officer in the perioperative area to ensure that guidelines are set forth according to the Occupational Safety and Health Administration, American National Standards Institute, and Association of periOperative Registered Nurses. This will promote the proper usage of the laser, ensure that precautions are taken, and confirm the maintenance of the different types of lasers.

Some types of lasers are:

- Carbon dioxide
- Argon
- Nd:YAG

Some basic guidelines for safety include:

- Laser warning signs specific to the type of laser being used posted at all entrances to the operating room
- Appropriate protective eyewear for personnel and patient that is applicable to the specific wavelength and optical density of the laser being used
- Windows covered, if applicable
- Calibration and testing of laser

- Use of smoke evacuator
- Fire extinguisher available
- Basin of water available in the operating room
- Wet towels on sterile field to drape patient and moist sponges during surgery
- Use water-soluble lubricants near the surgical site
- Anodized, dull, nonreflective, or matte-finish instruments used
- Laser placed in standby position when not being used

11

Surgical Instrumentation

Basic knowledge of surgical instruments and the usage of these instruments is important for the scrub nurse, certified surgical technologist, first assistant, and circulating nurse. To the novice, sometimes the instruments all look the same, and learning the names of each instrument is a daunting task.

During this part of your orientation, you will learn about:

- The general instrument categories
- Identification of differences in basic instruments
- The requirements for counting instruments
- Resolving count discrepancies

INSTRUMENT CATEGORIES

There are tens of thousands of instruments, and no one person can commit the name of each and every instrument to memory. The name of a particular instrument usually originates from one of the following:

- The inventor of the instrument
- The function of the instrument
- The appearance of the instrument
- The nickname of the instrument

In addition to the fact that many organizations and surgeons have personal names or even nicknames for some of the instruments, it may take a while to learn the technical names of each instrument. Therefore, instruments can be classified into these general categories by their usage:

- Cutting or dissecting
- Clamping or grasping
- Retracting
- Dilating or probing
- Laparoscopic
- Specialty

Most instruments are made of:

- Stainless steel (clamps)
- Tungsten carbide (scissors, needle holders)
- Aluminum (parts of instruments)
- Titanium (lightweight microsurgical instruments)

CUTTING OR DISSECTING INSTRUMENTS

These instruments are usually sharp and are used to cut through different types of tissue, such as:

- Skin
- Bone
- Ligaments/tendons

Some types of cutting or dissecting instruments include:

- Knives or scalpels
- Scissors
- Chisels/osteotomes (Figure 11.1)

Some basic types of scissors that are commonly used are:

- Metzenbaum
- Straight Mayo or suture scissors
- Curved Mayo
- Stevens

Scissors can be:

- Straight
- Curved
- Angular

The type of scissors used by the surgical team is dependent upon what it is being used for, where it is being used, and the surgeon's preference. Smaller scissors are commonly used on smaller patients

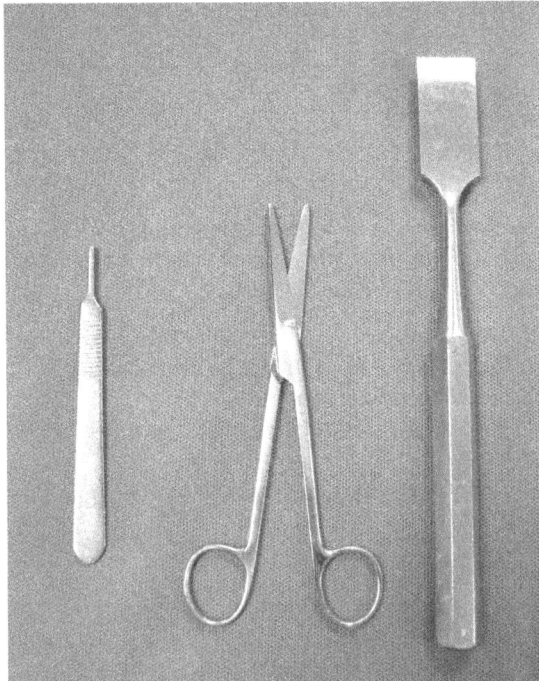

Figure 11.1 Knife handle (*left*), curved Mayo scissors (*middle*), and osteotome (*right*).

or smaller body parts, whereas longer or larger scissors are used on deeper or larger body parts.

Essential Facts

Only straight Mayo scissors should be used to cut sutures on the sterile field. When other scissors are used, it dulls the scissors blades and can loosen and/or separate the scissors at the screw joint. Therefore, each type of scissors should only be used for its specific intention.

CLAMPING OR GRASPING INSTRUMENTS

These instruments are used to:

- Occlude
- Grasp or hold

Some clamping or grasping instruments include:

- Clamp
- Dressing or tissue forceps
- Needle holder

Clamps

Clamps are abundant in the operating room, and the scrub personnel will have many different types of clamps on the sterile field.

Parts of the clamp are the following:

- Finger rings
- Shank (length varies depending on depth of wound)
- Ratchet (used to lock into place)
- Box lock, screw joint, or semibox (where the instrument joins together)
- Tip (varies depending on the type of clamp)

Figure 11.2 shows some of the most common basic clamps.

Forceps

Tissue can be grasped and held by instruments other than clamps, like forceps for example (Figure 11.3). These nonclamp graspers can have the following:

- A toothed end to grab tissue (e.g., skin)
- A nontoothed end to grab more delicate tissue (e.g., blood vessel)

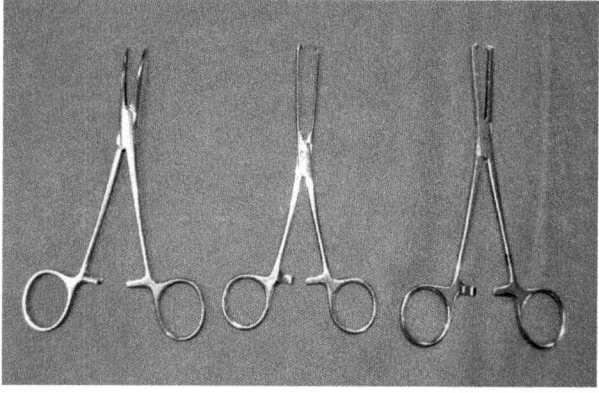

Figure 11.2 Curved Halstead (*left*), Allis (*middle*), and straight Kocher (*right*).

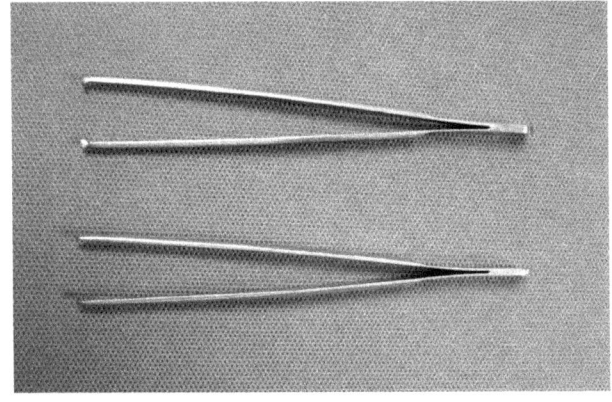

Figure 11.3 Mouse tooth forceps (*top*) and plain-tipped forceps (*bottom*).

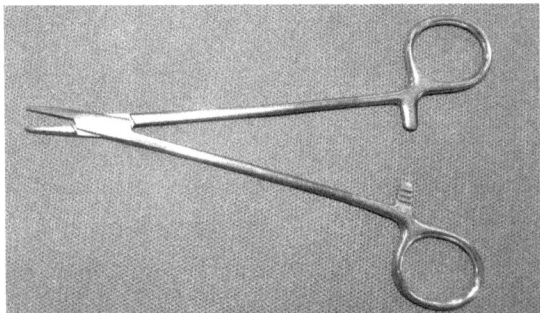

Figure 11.4 Needle holder.

Needle Holders

Needle holders (Figure 11.4) grasp surgical needles and have many different types of jaws. They may be ratcheted or nonratcheted depending on the following:

- Suture needle being held
- Tissue being sutured

RETRACTING INSTRUMENTS

These instruments can be used to:

- Hold open wound edges
- Hold structures aside
- Hold tissue aside for better visualization

Essential Facts

Question: Can you identify the instruments shown in Figure 11.5? Hint: Think of what category they fall into and try to start learning the instrument that way.

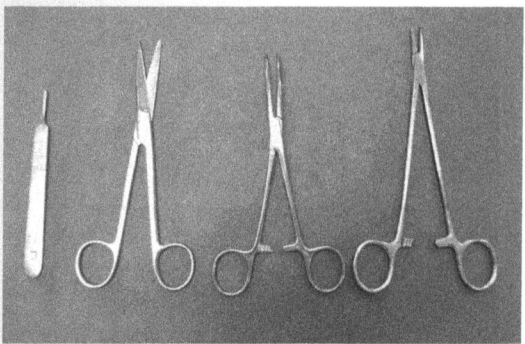

Figure 11.5

Answers: *Left to right:* Knife handle, straight Mayo scissors, Halstead clamp, needle holder.

Retractors can be manually held or can be self-retaining, which means they do not require a person to hold them in place (Figure 11.6). Some basic retractors include:

- Army–navy (manually held)
- Vein (manually held)
- Richardson (manually held)
- Weitlaner (self-retaining)
- Balfour (self-retaining)

DILATING OR PROBING INSTRUMENTS

Dilators are used to stretch or enlarge a natural opening or orifice. Some common dilators are:

- Hank/Hegar dilators (used on the cervix; Figure 11.7)
- Urethral dilators
- Vascular dilators
- Tracheal dilators

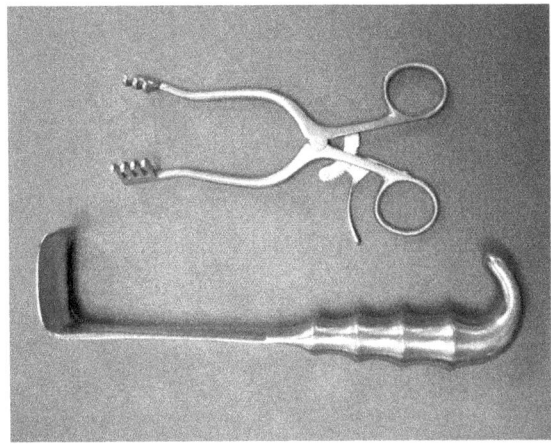

Figure 11.6 Retractors: Weitlaner (self-retaining; *top*); Richardson (manually held; *bottom*).

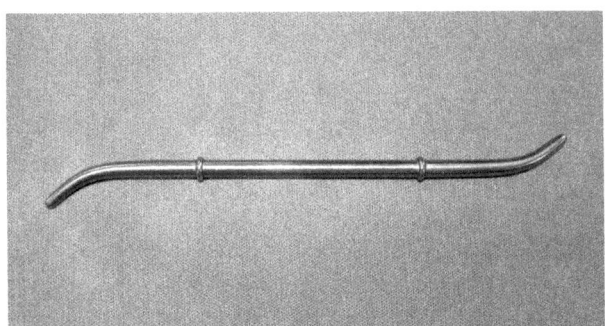

Figure 11.7 Hank dilator.

Probes

Probes can be rigid or malleable. They are used to explore, to dilate, or to gently move structures depending upon where the probe is used.

Some common probes include:

- Silver probe (goes with the grooved director; Figure 11.8)
- Lacrimal probe
- Fistula probe
- Laparoscopic probe

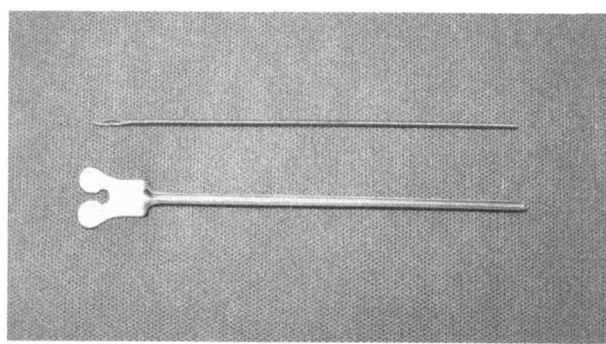

Figure 11.8 Silver probe (*top*) and groove director (*bottom*).

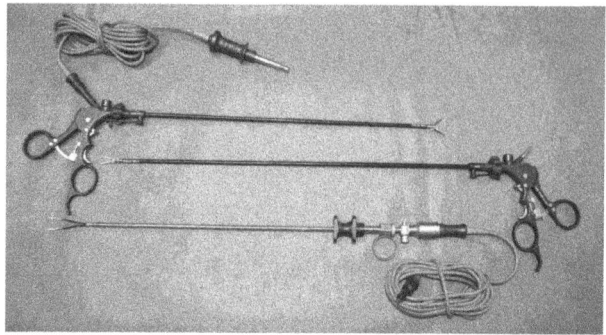

Figure 11.9 Laparoscopic dissector (*top*), grasper (*middle*), and Kleppinger forceps (*bottom*).

LAPAROSCOPIC INSTRUMENTS

Laparoscopic instruments can be disposable, resposable, or reusable. They commonly have the following parts:

- Handle
- Sheath
- Tip

The laparoscopic instruments must pass through the trocar and can come in varying diameters from 3 to 12 mm. A comparable-size trocar must be used.

Some common basic laparoscopic instruments are the following:

- Dissector (Figure 11.9)
- Scissors
- Grasper (Figure 11.9)
- Kleppinger forceps (Figure 11.9)

SPECIALTY INSTRUMENTS

Various specialty instruments can be used depending on the surgical specialty. These instruments should be learned when rotating through each surgical specialty.

Some specialty instruments are the following:

- Saws
- Drills
- Elevators
- Muscle biopsy needles and cannulas
- Awls

Essential Facts

When scrubbed, if you are worried about remembering the name of a few of the instruments, you can get a sterile marking pen and write the names next to the instruments on the paper drape. It is not recommended to use this technique all the time or as a replacement for learning the names, but it can be used when necessary to help reinforce the names.

REQUIREMENTS FOR COUNTING INSTRUMENTS

The risk of retained surgical items (RSIs) is a very serious situation for the patient, the entire surgical team, and the hospital. Many states require this event to be publically reported, meaning that the public has a heightened awareness of this issue and the information can be viewed by anyone. Federal and state agencies, accrediting bodies, third-party payers, and professional organizations consider RSIs to be a sentinel or "never" event. The risk for RSIs can increase with:

- Emergent surgery
- Unexpected change in procedure
- Multiple procedures
- High body mass index
- Communication breakdown

It is an important standard practice to count all surgical instruments and keep all instrumentation in the operating room until the patient has left the room.

The risk of RSI can be limited by:

- Having standardized instrument trays
- Using preprinted count sheets
- Using only even numbers of instruments, if possible
- Creating and following clear processes each and every time
- Multidisciplinary teamwork

Counts must be performed:

- Before the surgical procedure (initial count)
- When instruments are added to the sterile field
- Before closure of a cavity within a cavity (only for soft items[1])
- At wound closure (final count)
- Upon permanent relief of scrub personnel

The approved methods of counting instruments are:

- Aloud
- Between both the scrub and circulator
- Concurrently viewing instruments by both the scrub and circulator
- Separating each instrument and counting each one
- Identifying and accounting for multiple pieces
- Progressing in a logical order (from field, to mayo stand, to back table)

Resolving Count Discrepancies

A count discrepancy occurs when the quantity of instruments started with does not reflect the quantity of instruments finished with, or when an instrument becomes broken or separated into parts.

In such case, it is important to:

- Notify the surgeon and perioperative team members.
- Inspect the surgical wound.
- Search the sterile field.
- Search the surrounding areas in the operating room (including under the operating room bed, in drapes, in the garbage).
- Obtain an x-ray film of the surgical wound.
- Follow specific hospital policy and procedures.
- Document variant findings.

---

[1] Soft items include sponges, towels, sharps, and miscellaneous items. This does not include instruments.

Adjunct Count Technology

There are many new technologies that assist in the counting of instruments in the operating room. Such technology devices include:

- Bar coding
- Radiofrequency identification
- Radiofrequency hybrid

These devices do not take away from exemplary nursing practice. Adjunct technology should be used as an additional measure of safety for verification of count accuracy in conjunction with manual counting and standardized procedures.

12

Electrosurgery

The electrosurgery unit is one of the most utilized and valued pieces of equipment in the operating room. Therefore, it is imperative that all members of the surgical team understand how it should be properly used to minimize the potential for injury to both the patient and the surgical team.

During this part of your orientation, you will learn about:

- Components of the electrosurgery unit (ESU)
- Methods of electrosurgery
- Different tissue effects
- ESU settings and hand pieces
- Safety considerations
- The need for smoke evacuation

The ESU provides high-frequency electrical current to tissue to:

- Remove lesions
- Stop bleeding
- Cut tissue
- Vaporize tissue

COMPONENTS OF THE ESU

The ESU consists of:

- Generator (ESU machine)
- Active electrode (hand piece)
- Return electrode (ground pad)

METHODS OF ELECTROSURGERY

- Monopolar
- Bipolar
- Ultrasonic
- Argon-enhanced coagulation
- Vessel sealing

Monopolar

Monopolar electrosurgery is the most common method. To complete a circuit, the generator will produce the electron flow and voltage to the active electrode through the patient, then to the ground pad, and then back to the generator (Figure 12.1).

The ground pad or return electrode removes the current from the patient and brings it back to the generator. When the energy is concentrated to a small area, such as the electrode tip, the tissue provides resistance, also known as *impedance*. This resistance produces heat.

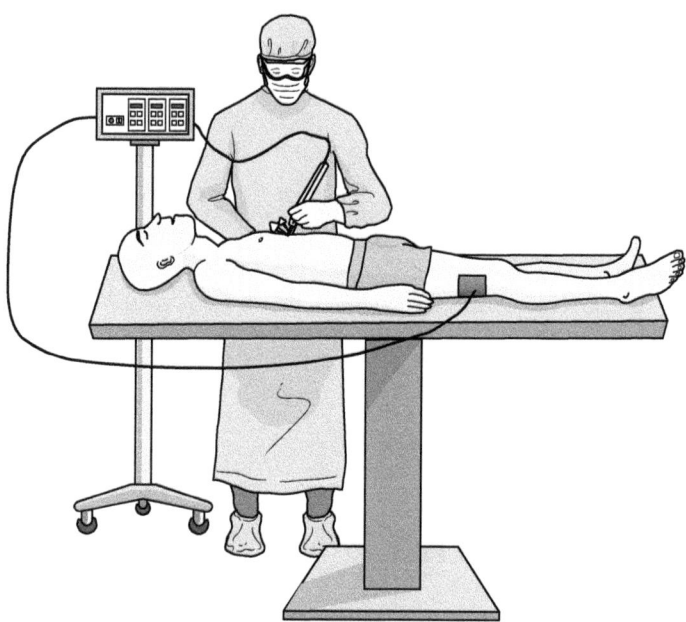

Figure 12.1 Monopolar circuit.

Ground Pad (Return Electrode)

Use of a return electrode monitoring (REM) ground pad is recommended. REM ground pads monitor the amount of impedance, or amount of voltage required to push the electrons through the tissue at the patient-pad site, and will deactivate the generator prior to injury. These pads prevent patient burns resulting from inadequate contact of the return electrode. (There are still non-REM pads available on the market, and these should be used with extreme caution.)

Ground Pad Placement and Considerations

The ground pad should be:

- Placed as close as possible to the surgical site
- Positioned on a well-vascularized muscle (e.g., thigh, flank, buttocks)
- Changed immediately if it gets wet from fluid or prep solution
- Always used in adherence with patient weight guidelines (they come in many sizes—neonate, pediatric, adult)

The Do Nots of ground pads are:

- Do not place the ground pad so that it overlaps onto itself.
- Do not place it over bony areas, tattoos, scars, or metal implants.
- Do not take the pad out until application (it can dry out).
- Do not plug the ground pad in until it is placed on the patient.
- Do not cut or alter the ground pad in any way.

Return Electrode (Ground Pad) Burns

A burn may result if the temperature at the return electrode site becomes too hot. Therefore, proper placement of the return electrode and constant monitoring to ensure that the return electrode is not compromised are important. Certain situations can increase the potential for burns, such as:

- Excessive hair
- Adipose tissue
- Bony prominences
- Fluid
- Adhesive failure
- Scar tissue
- Tattoos
- Irregular body contour

> **Essential Facts**
>
> **Question:** An elderly malnourished patient is scheduled for a hysterectomy. Upon the preoperative assessment, you find out that she broke her right hip 3 years ago and a prosthetic was used to stabilize the right hip. What would the proper placement be for the return electrode (ground pad)?
>
> **Answer:** It should be placed as close as possible to the surgical site, on a well-vascularized area that is free from scar and metal. Therefore, the left thigh would be appropriate if, when examined, it meets the criteria. Other options are possibly the arm, flank, or left buttock.

Bipolar Circuit

Bipolar electrosurgery is commonly used in ophthalmic and vascular surgery, and when a patient has an implanted electronic device (IED). There is no grounding pad and the tines (prongs) on the bipolar forceps are the active electrode and return electrode (Figure 12.2).

Therefore, to complete a circuit, the generator will produce the electron flow and voltage to the active electrode through the patient, then back to the opposing tine of the instrument, and then back to the generator.

Foot Pedal

A foot pedal can be utilized for the ESU when hand activation is not available. This requires plugging in the proper foot pedal and placing the pedal at the surgeon's foot. Be certain to make the surgeon aware

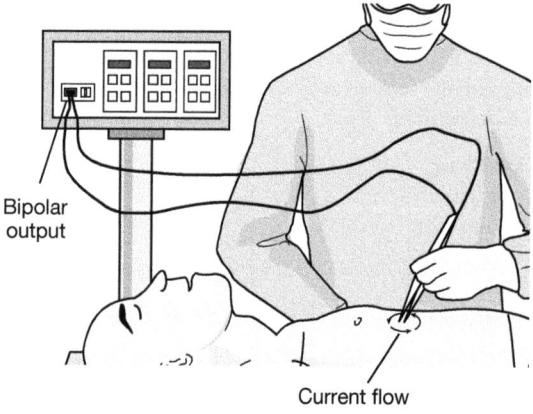

Figure 12.2 Bipolar circuit.

of the placement of the foot pedal to prevent unintentional activation of the electrocautery unit.

Ultrasonic Radiofrequency

Ultrasonic radiofrequency uses alternating current to create friction at high temperatures to cause coagulation or ablation. (Refer to Chapter 13 for more detailed information.)

Argon-Enhanced Electrosurgery

Argon-enhanced electrosurgery uses argon gas to increase the effectiveness of the ESU, resulting in less tissue damage and less blood loss. This method is monopolar and requires the use of a ground pad. This method is commonly used for obtaining hemostasis over large surface areas (e.g., in radical oncology procedures).

Vessel-Sealing Instruments

These are instruments that can seal tissue and vessels up to approximately 7 mm with heat as opposed to using sutures. The vessel-sealing device can be used on open or laparoscopic surgical procedures. This method is bipolar and therefore does not require a ground pad. The energy flows from the generator, to the device, out of one of the tines, through the tissue, back into the opposing tine of the instrument, and then back to the generator.

Essential Facts

Question: The surgeon decides to use the bipolar cautery. What equipment would you need to get?
Answer: You will need the ESU generator, bipolar hand piece, and cord. If the bipolar hand piece is foot activated, then a foot pedal will also be needed and should be attached to the generator.

DIFFERENT TISSUE EFFECTS

The ESU can provide different tissue effects depending upon the type of tip, the tissue, and how the tip is used. The different tissue effects (Figure 12.3) are as follows:

- Cutting and vaporizing (uses high heat)
- Coagulation (uses less heat)
- Desiccation (when the electrode comes in direct contact with the tissue)
- Fulguration (less heat and more coagulation disseminated over a wide area to char the tissue)

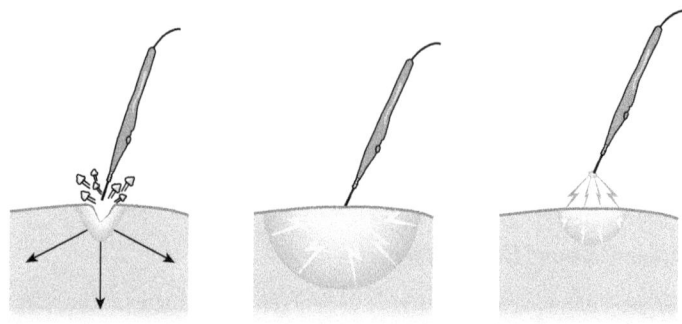

Figure 12.3 Electrosurgical cutting (*left*), desiccation (*middle*), and fulguration (*right*).

ESU SETTINGS

The generator can be set to deliver different amounts of power depending on the surgeon's preference, the tissue type, and the tissue effect that is desired. The settings will vary within these main categories:

- Cutting (100% on)
- Blend I (50% on and 50% off)
- Blend II (40% on and 60% off)
- Blend III (25% on and 75% off)
- Coagulation (6% on and 94% off)

Cutting produces the most heat, whereas coagulation produces much less heat and instead of vaporizing the tissue, it coagulates the tissue. The blend I to III options are not a combination of cutting and coagulating, but the application of heat on and off to produce varying tissue effects.

Power Settings on the ESU

The ESU power settings can range from 1 to 100 watts, and commonly depend on the following:

- Desired tissue effect
- Size and type of active electrode tip
- Duration of activation of generator
- Surgeon's manipulation of the active electrode

ESU Hand-Piece Tips

There are many different types of tips that can be placed on the hand piece. Some common tips are:

- Blade tip
- Needle tip
- Ball tip
- Loop tip

The tips can also have different finishes that help prevent tissue from accumulating and reducing the effect of the tip. Some such finishes are:

- Coated tips
- Teflon tips
- Guarded tips

Essential Facts

Because there are so many different variations in types of tips and finishes, it is important to always use a standardized premade tip. It is not recommended to make your own tip by cutting catheters and placing them over a premade tip. This can potentially be hazardous and unsafe.

Cleaning the ESU Tips

The ESU tip can accumulate debris, char, and excess tissue. This is known as *eschar*. The ESU tip should be cleaned often for proper functionality. It is important to check the tip and clean it with one of the following:

- The tip cleaner (a nonabrasive pad made for this purpose)
- A wet 4 × 4 x-ray-detectable sponge (recommended for Teflon and coated tips)

SAFETY CONSIDERATIONS

The ESU is a very effective piece of equipment, but safety is paramount whenever using this device. It is important to:

- Keep the active electrode in a nonconductive holder to prevent accidental activation.
- Keep a moist sponge and water/saline solution available on the sterile field in case of fire when using the ESU.

- Use the lowest effective power settings.
- Use the bipolar ESU when the patient has an ICD or pacemaker.
- Check the insulation for integrity, especially reusable cords. Small holes in the insulation can cause a burn; this is referred to as *insulation failure*.

The Do Nots of ESU safety:

- Do not activate the ESU in the presence of flammable agents (e.g., prep solutions that have not dried, oxygen).
- Do not place anything, especially liquids, on top of the generator.
- Do not wrap the cord of the active electrode around any metal instrument, or bunch it together with other cords.

There are other safety concerns that can occur when performing laparoscopic surgery and using the ESU. These include:

- Direct coupling
- Capacitive coupling
- Alternate-site burns (can occur laparoscopically or with open procedure)

Direct Coupling

This occurs when the tip of the active electrode comes in contact with another metal instrument or anything that conducts electricity. An example of this would be faulty insulation on the active electrode and the current that comes out at that point causes burning to whatever it is touching.

Capacitive Coupling

This occurs when an active electrode induces stray current to a conductor through insulation. An example of this would be an insulated electrode surrounded by a metal trocar with a plastic screw. This would set up currents between two conductors with an insulator in between.

Alternate-Site Burns

Alternate-site burns occur when the current from a grounded ESU generator does not return to the generator and goes to an alternate ground site. This can result in a burn. An example of this is seen when the monopolar active electrode is activated and instead of the current returning back to the ground pad, it goes to the ECG electrode.

EVACUATION OF SURGICAL SMOKE

When tissue is vaporized by the ESU the by-product is surgical smoke. Literature discloses that surgical smoke:

- Is a carcinogen
- Contains viral DNA and bacteria
- Contains toxic gases and vapor (e.g., benzene, formaldehyde)
- Is a possible irritant

Precaution must be taken to prevent the inhalation of surgical smoke by the perioperative team and patient. The Association of periOperative Registered Nurses recommends the use of a smoke evacuation system for all surgical procedures that require the use of the ESU, including ultrasonic procedures. This is also required for laser procedures and applies to both open and laparoscopic surgery.

There are many products on the market that evacuate smoke with high-efficiency filters. The smoke evacuator system can be one of the following:

- Handheld device
- Device that attaches to the ESU tip
- Device that attaches to a trocar

The smell of surgical smoke permeates the air quickly at a concentration rate of about 60,000 to 1 million particles per cubic foot within 5 minutes of ESU usage.

13

Surgical Energy and Stapling Devices

The operating room is full of many different energy and stapling devices. These devices provide quick and precise energy and stapling for the surgeon to employ throughout any surgical procedure. Energy devices can control bleeding and seal off vessels, and stapling devices can accurately cut and place a line of staples. It is important for the scrub nurse, certified surgical technologist, RN first assistant, and circulating nurse to know exactly how to use each device safely and to understand the differences among these devices.

During this part of your orientation, you will learn about:

- Different types of surgical energy
- Different tissue effects
- Settings, hand pieces, and tips
- Safety considerations
- Different types of stapling devices

DIFFERENT TYPES OF SURGICAL ENERGY

There are many different types of surgical energy, including:

- Ultrasonic
- Advanced bipolar
- Radiofrequency
- Cryoablation
- Microwave ablation

Ultrasonic Surgical Energy

This is an ultrasonic wave that moves through tissue at a rate of 55,000 vibrations per second or a frequency of 55,000 Hz. This very high vibration will cut, coagulate, and cavitate tissue. *Cavitation* is the vaporization of tissue by removing the liquid from the tissue, and expanding the tissue plane for dissection. Therefore, the energy flows from the generator to the hand piece, then to the tissue. Ultrasonic surgical energy provides slow and controllable heat with less tissue damage than the electrosurgery unit (ESU). It can be used on open and laparoscopic procedures.

Components of Ultrasonic Surgical Energy

- Generator
- Hand piece
- Blade/tip
- Foot pedal (if not hand activated)

Ultrasonic energy is affected by:

- Time in contact with tissue
- Blade pressure
- Tissue tension and placement
- Power level

Generator settings for different tissue effects:

- Power level 1 (increased coagulation)
- Power level 2
- Power level 3 (usually the preset setting)
- Power level 4
- Power level 5 (increased cutting)

Safety considerations include:

- Checking for small cracks in the hand piece and cord (especially if reusable)
- Checking blade placement
- Watching for overheating (generator will turn off)
- Listening for warning signal if pressure on tissue is too high

Different blades/tips (Figure 13.1) are:

- Blade
- Hook
- Shears

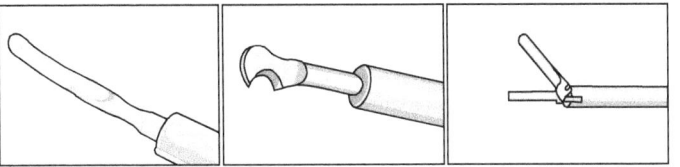

Figure 13.1 *Left to right:* blade, hook, shears.

Common surgical procedures that use ultrasonic energy are:

- Sleeve gastrectomy
- Laparoscopic cholecystectomy
- Laparoscopic hysterectomy

Essential Facts

Question: The surgeon decides that ultrasonic energy is required for the patient undergoing a cholecystectomy. What should you bring into the operating room?

Answer: You should bring the generator, hand piece, blade/tip that the surgeon prefers, and foot pedal (if not hand activated).

Advanced Bipolar Energy

Similar to regular bipolar energy, the energy flows from the generator to the instrument, to the tissue, and back through the opposing jaw to return to the generator.

Components of advanced bipolar energy are:

- Generator
- Cord (if not connected to the hand piece)
- Hand piece
- Foot pedal (if not hand activated)

It will seal vessels by:

- Cutting
- Coagulating

Advanced bipolar energy has these characteristics:

- It has low voltage.
- It seals vessels up to approximately 7 mm.
- It is able to accurately measure and control electrical current on tissue.
- It has current that is pulsed.

In advanced bipolar energy, generator settings do not vary. It uses one setting that will heat up to 100°C. Also, no ground pad is required because it is bipolar.

Safety considerations include:

- Checking for small cracks in the hand piece or cord (especially if reusable)
- Checking blade placement
- Checking for electromagnetic interference with other equipment (may have to move away from other devices, such as ESU)

Different blades/tips are:

- Blade with jaws
- Articulating and rotating blades

Common surgical procedures that use advanced bipolar energy include:

- Hysterectomy
- Tubal ligation
- Colon resection

Radiofrequency Surgical Energy

This is the surgical use of low-frequency radio waves through electrodes to cause friction and an increased tissue temperature.

Components of radiofrequency (RF) energy are:

- Generator
- Cord (bipolar or monopolar)
- Hand piece
- Tip
- Plate
- Foot pedal (if not hand activated)

The plate is a return path for the radio waves and is placed on the patient.

Essential Facts

Caution should be taken when using any energy device for a patient with a pacemaker or implantable cardioverter defibrillator (ICD). The surgical energy may cause the pacemaker or ICD to malfunction or may possibly damage the device. Therefore, it is important for the surgeon and anesthesia provider to know that the patient

(continued)

(*continued*)

> has a pacemaker or ICD before using surgical energy. Most often the pacemaker or ICD will be switched into a different mode by a company representative during surgery.

This low-temperature RF energy will:

- Cut
- Coagulate
- Fulgurate
- Have bipolar capability

Safety considerations include:

- Checking for small cracks in the hand piece, cord, and plate (especially if reusable)
- Making certain that the correct hand piece is connected to the correct cord

Different hand pieces include:

- Monopolar
- Bipolar
- Blade

Different tips that can be attached to these hand pieces are:

- Regular
- Fine
- Superfine

They also come in straight, angled, and loop.

Common surgical procedures that use RF surgical energy include:

- Eye surgery
- Nasal surgery to reduce turbinates
- Tonsillectomy
- Cardiac ablation for arrhythmias

Cryoablation

This is the use of extreme cold to destroy tissue.

Components of cryoablation energy are:

- Generator
- Cord (if not connected to the hand piece)
- Hand piece
- Foot pedal (if not hand activated)

It can be used to:

- Dissect tissue
- Ablate tissue
- Occlude tissue

Because it can be used for so many different surgical procedures, the settings vary. Safety considerations include:

- Checking for small cracks in the hand piece and cord (especially if reusable)
- Checking blade placement

Common surgical procedures that use cryoablation energy are:

- Cardiac ablation
- Eye surgery
- Uterine ablation

Microwave Ablation

This is the use of a microwave antenna that is placed directly into a tumor. The heat from the microwaves destroys cells and tissue. Microwave ablation can reach high temperatures to destroy large tumors. The microwave frequency is approximately 900 MHz.

Components of microwave ablation are:

- Generator
- Cord (if not connected to a hand piece)
- Hand piece
- Foot pedal (if not hand activated)

Generator settings vary depending on the tumor.

This treatment can be done:

- Percutaneously (needle-like puncture through the skin)
- Laparoscopically
- Open

Safety considerations include:

- Checking for small cracks in the hand piece and cord (especially if reusable)
- Checking for electromagnetic interference with other equipment (may have to move away from other devices, such as ESU)

Common surgical procedures that use microwave ablation include:

- Cancer treatment for liver tumor
- Cancer treatment for colorectal tumor

DIFFERENT TYPES OF STAPLING DEVICES

Staplers provide a quick way to cut and staple tissue. They come in all different shapes and sizes; choice of staple type is dependent on:

- Tissue thickness
- Type of tissue
- Patient anatomy
- Surgeon preference

Stapling devices provide:

- Compression
- Hemostasis through staple line
- Cutting of tissue

Staples are commonly made of titanium or stainless steel and do not dissolve.

Essential Facts

Because surgical staples are made of metal, it is important to inform a patient that staples were used during surgery. If the patient ever undergoes magnetic resonance imaging (MRI), they will be questioned regarding metal in the body. Surgical staples can be affected by MRI, but rest assured because most staples are made of titanium, they usually are not a problem.

Common types of staplers and types of tissue that they are used on are:

- Straight cutters—for use across tissue (e.g., colon resection)
- Circular—for use within the gastrointestinal tract (e.g., hemorrhoid or lower anterior resection)
- Curved—for lower pelvic access (e.g., lower anterior resection)
- Linear cutters— or use across tissue for open procedures (e.g., wedge resection, colon resection)

Reloads

Reloads are the cartridges placed in the stapling device each time it is fired. The reloads will have staples of a specific size and shape. Each device can only be fired or used a specific number of times, which is set by the manufacturer.

Safety considerations for stapling devices:

- Only use the reloads according to the manufacturer's directions, meaning that if the stapler fires five times, only use it up to five times.
- Be certain to clean the jaws of the stapler device in saline or water before reloading; leftover staples will jam the device.
- Only use reloads that are meant for the device.

Hemoclips and Multifeed Stapling Devices

Hemoclips are single clips that can be used on vessels to stop bleeding. They can come in a multifeed device that can deploy consecutive staples.

Hemoclips commonly come in three sizes:

- Small
- Medium
- Large

Other multifeed stapling devices are used to staple mesh or secure soft tissue. These types of devices are commonly used to staple and secure mesh during hernia surgery. This can be accomplished during an open hernia repair or laparoscopically.

Multifeed stapling devices commonly come in the following sizes:

- 4-mm staples
- 4.8-mm staples

14

Surgical Dressings

Surgical dressings are applied at the end of the surgical procedure over the surgical wound before the drapes are removed. Once the drapes are removed, the dressing is secured in place. There are many choices of surgical dressings as well as products used to secure the dressings to the patient.

During this part of your orientation, you will learn about:

- Surgical wound classifications and types of wound closure
- The purpose of surgical dressings
- Different types of dressings and other related products
- Products to secure the dressing
- Casting materials

SURGICAL WOUND CLASSIFICATIONS

Surgical wound classifications are determined by the Centers for Disease Control and Prevention (CDC), and there are four different wound classifications:

- Class 1: Clean wounds (uninfected operative wound in which no inflammation is encountered)
- Class 2: Clean/contaminated wounds (respiratory, alimentary, genital, or urinary tracts are entered under controlled conditions and without unusual contamination)
- Class 3: Contaminated wounds (operations with major breaks in sterile technique or gross spillage from the gastrointestinal

tract, and incisions in which acute, nonpurulent inflammation is encountered)
- Class 4: Dirty or infected wounds (old traumatic wounds with retained devitalized tissue and those that involve existing clinical infection or perforated viscera)

These classifications indicate the probability of an infection. Therefore, the higher the number, the greater chance that an infection may occur.

Essential Facts

Question: A dilatation and curettage is scheduled. What wound classification would this procedure fall under?
Answer: A dilatation and curettage enters the genital tract and is considered a Class 2 procedure.

Dressings can be placed over all four classes of wounds, but sometimes a wound is left undressed or open, which can benefit healing by:

- Allowing the wound to be observed
- Rendering the wound easier to clean
- Lessening adhesive skin reaction from tape
- Providing more comfort for the patient

TYPES OF WOUND CLOSURE

Wounds close in different ways. There are three main types of wound closure:

- Primary intention: Edges of wounds are closed by sutures or staples
- Secondary intention or granulation: Wound is left open and heals from the bottom up
- Tertiary intention or delayed primary: Wound is left open initially and then closed by primary intention a few days later

PURPOSE OF SURGICAL DRESSINGS

When dressings are used, their purposes include:

- To protect the wound
- To absorb drainage from the wound

- To cushion, support, splint, or immobilize the wound
- To provide hemostasis and minimize dead space
- To prevent infection

DIFFERENT TYPES OF SURGICAL DRESSINGS AND PRODUCTS

Types of dressings are listed and described in Table 14.1.

Table 14.1

Types of Dressings

Product	Material	Usage
Cotton gauze abdominal (4 × 4)	Woven cotton	Common for wounds
Kling Webril	Woven/nonwoven cotton roll	Common for extremities
Telfa	Nonadherent gauze pad	Placed on incision to prevent dressing from adhering
Steri-Strips	Adhesive strips	Common in plastic surgery
Drain sponge	Woven cotton	Placed around drain site
Vaseline gauze	Nonadherent gauze impregnated with Vaseline	Commonly used to pack a wound
Adaptic	Nonadherent dressing of cellulose acetate coated with silicone	Used on many types of wounds
Xeroform	3% bismuth tribromophenate and petrolatum	Common on orthopedic wounds
Gauze packing	Various-sized packing	Can be used to pack a wound
Lodoform packing	Various-sized impregnated antiseptic	Can be used to pack a wound
Tegaderm (OpSite)	Transparent film	Commonly placed over intravenous lines
Duoderm	Hydrocolloid	Used if wound is exposed to moisture
Biopatch	Foam	Absorbent, can be used on central lines

Table 14.2

Products to Secure the Dressing

Product	Material	Usage
Paper tape	Paper	To secure dressings
Cloth tape	Cotton cloth	To secure dressings
Silk tape	Silk	To secure dressings
Adhesive tape	Plastic	Common over eye dressing
Elastic adhesive tape	High-twist, woven cotton	Supportive and common for extremity
Abdominal binder	Knit elastic and Velcro	Nondisposable, used after abdominal surgery for pressure
Montgomery straps	Adhesive straps	Used for frequent dressing changes

SECURING THE DRESSING

After the dressing is placed at the end of the surgery and the drapes are removed, the dressing must then be secured in place. At this point, the surgeon or another member of the perioperative team will remove their gown and gloves and secure the dressing in place. There are many products that can be used to secure the dressing (Table 14.2). Most of them are hypoallergenic and latex free.

Essential Facts

Montgomery straps are commonly used by nurses for frequent dressing changes because they preserve the skin's integrity. Because Montgomery straps stay on for a few days, this eliminates the need to reapply tape each time the dressing needs to be changed. This prevents skin breakdown. Montgomery straps can be secured with twill ties, cut gauze, safety pins, or other tying materials.

OTHER PRODUCTS FOR WOUNDS

Wound VACs

Wound VACs create a negative pressure on wounds that are difficult to heal and do not respond positively to traditional dressings.

Wound VACs are commonly applied in the operating room at the end of the surgical procedure or after a wound is debrided.

The typical components of a wound VAC are:

- VAC pump machine
- Cartridge to collect drainage
- Dressing sponge (comes in many sizes)

Silver-Impregnated Dressings

Silver-impregnated dressings are topical antimicrobial dressings that contain silver and may be used to prevent or manage infection. They come in a variety of shapes and sizes.

Soft Silicone-Bordered Dressings

Soft silicone-bordered dressings can contain three or five layers and are used as a component of pressure ulcer prevention in patients who are at high risk of pressure ulcers in the operating room (OR). They come in different sizes and are applied prior to surgery on any area that can potentially develop a pressure ulcer (i.e., sacrum; Fulbrook, Mbuzi, & Miles, 2019).

Skin Substitutes

Sometimes instead of performing a split-thickness skin graft to cover a wound, a skin substitute can be used to cover the wound.

Skin substitutes can be

- Live tissue (e.g., Apligraf)
- Nonliving tissue (e.g., Integra)
- Synthetic tissue (e.g., Biobrane)

Essential Facts

It is important to consider the religious beliefs of all patients. Therefore, the perioperative team should have a greater understanding of religious views and, during the informed consent procedure, should include a discussion about animal-derived surgical implants or products to avoid religious distress and possible litigation. For example, persons of Jewish, Muslim, and Hindu faiths many not want porcine and bovine surgical products used as treatment options.

The type of skin substitute is dependent upon:

- Surgeon preference
- Location of wound

- Type of wound
- Manufacturer's approved uses and indications for product

It is important to remember that some of these products may be derived from animals and can conflict with certain religious and cultural beliefs.

Growth Factors

Growth factors may be injected or placed topically onto wounds to promote healing. Growth factors are proteins such as cytokines and peptides. These proteins stimulate cell growth.

Some common growth factors are:

- Epidermal growth factor
- Keratinocyte growth factor
- Vascular endothelial growth factor

CASTING

A cast can be placed on an extremity or portion of the body to support, splint, and/or immobilize it.

Casting material can be:

- Plaster
- Fiberglass

Casting material comes in many different sizes. Some common sizes are:

- 3 to 4 inch (e.g., on arm)
- 5 to 6 inch (e.g., on leg)

Usually, the smaller the extremity, the smaller the casting material, and the larger the extremity, the larger the casting material.

Application of a Cast

To apply a cast, several items are needed, including:

- Cast padding (soft material to go against the patient's skin)
- Waterproof cast padding (so that the cast can get wet)
- Stockinette
- Cast material (either plaster or fiberglass)
- Lukewarm water (used to soak cast material to soften and mold)

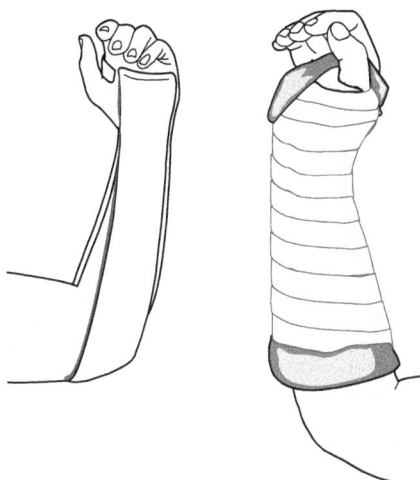

Figure 14.1 Splint application.

Splints

A splint is a partial cast. A splint may be used if there is swelling, but provides less support than a cast. In order to apply a splint, several items are needed. A splint can be made of plaster, fiberglass, or metal (common for fingers).

Application of a Splint

To apply a splint (Figure 14.1), several items are needed. These items can include:

- Cast padding
- Stockinette
- Ace bandage
- Casting material or roll of splint material, which can be cut to individual lengths; or metal splint
- Lukewarm water (not needed for metal splint)

Reference

Fulbrook, P., Mbuzi, V., & Miles, S. (2019). Effectiveness of prophylactic sacral protective dressings to prevent pressure injury: A systematic review and meta-analysis. *International journal of nursing studies, 100*, 103400.

IV

Additional Operating Room Considerations

15

Medications

The operating room is a medication-intensive setting. It is important to establish safety processes on and off the sterile field to prevent medication errors. Medication errors in the United States have affected at least 7 million people every year, resulting in 7,000 to 9,000 deaths in the United States annually (Tariq, Vashisht, Sinha, & Scherbak, 2021).

During this part of your orientation, you will learn about:

- Preparing medications
- Transferring medications onto the sterile field
- Handling and administering medications on the sterile field
- Disposing of medications
- Handling of chemotherapy agents

PREPARING MEDICATIONS (DRUG COMPOUNDING)

The American Pharmacists Association defines *drug compounding* as the mixing of ingredients, including dilution, admixture (mixing of medications), repackaging, reconstitution, and other manipulations of sterile products, to prepare a medication for patient use. Many institutions recommend that sterile medications should be prepared by the pharmacy, unless it is an emergency situation. The administration of the final compounded products must begin within 1 hour of preparation.

To comply with these safety regulations, operating rooms should be using:

- Ready-to-use medications, which can be compounded in the pharmacy or offsite
- Standardized dosing, whereby medications and concentrations are provided in set amounts
- Automated dispensing devices, which can help control and reduce error, but do not eliminate error
- Notifications for high-alert medications, and also providing notifications to all staff regarding confusing names of medications

High-alert medications are medications that bear a heightened risk of causing significant patient harm if administered. The Institute for Safe Medication Practices (ISMP) lists several medications that fall within this category.

Some high-alert medications include:

- Adrenergic agonists, administered intravenously (epinephrine)
- Moderate sedation agents, administered intravenously (midazolam)
- Neuromuscular blocking agents (succinylcholine)
- Sodium chloride for injection (> 0.9% concentration)

Confusing Names

Confusing the names of medications presents another potential for error. The ISMP has also issued a list of confusing drug names that include look-alike and sound-alike medications. The ISMP recommends bolded tall man (uppercase) letters to help draw attention to the dissimilarities in look-alike drug names (ISMP, 2019).

Some look-alike and sound-alike medications include:

- **DOP**amine/**DOBUT**amine
- Fenta**NYL**/**SUF**entanil
- predni**SONE**/predniso**LONE**

TRANSFERRING OF MEDICATIONS

When transferring medications onto the sterile field, it is important to create a safe process that is adhered to and consistently practiced each and every time. This will prevent the risk of contamination and the possibility of recording information incorrectly when labeling medications. Transferring of medication is twofold and involves the circulating RN and the scrub RN or certified surgical technologist (CST).

The role of the circulating RN includes:

- Using a transfer device (e.g., spike, filter straw, needle, and syringe) to transfer medications from the vial/ampule to the sterile field; pouring medications increases the risk of contamination
- Ensuring that stoppers are not removed from vials
- Examining medication for particles or discoloration and ensuring that they are not used if compromised
- Checking expiration dates
- Transferring only one medication at a time
- Confirming dose limits of each particular medication with the surgeon
- Confirming medication name, strength, dose, and expiration date with the scrub RN/CST

The role of the scrub RN or CST includes:

- Labeling the container immediately upon receiving the medication
- Ensuring that the label includes, at minimum, the name of the medication, strength, and concentration
- Confirming the label with the circulating nurse
- If the medication is being transferred to another container (e.g., syringe), ensure that the new container is labeled in the same manner as the previous one
- Ensuring that any unlabeled medication on the sterile field is discarded

Essential Facts

Sterile water and normal saline are also considered medications and must be labeled on the sterile field. Most medications are clear liquids and can easily be misidentified. Even if normal saline is the only medication on the field, it must be labeled each and every time.

HANDLING AND ADMINISTRATION OF MEDICATIONS ON THE STERILE FIELD

Surgical procedures can become hurried at different points during the procedure, and it is important to always handle medications with caution. Acquire and use a clear communication process during the procedure and adhere to this process to decrease the chance of any potential medication error.

Handling and administrating medications should include:

- Clear communication regarding, at minimum, the name and strength of the medication when passing it to the surgeon or any other member of the surgical team
- The verification of all medications when staff members are being relieved for a break or at the end of the shift
- The use of proper containers in order not to compromise the medication (e.g., plastic cup would be acceptable)
- Verification that medications that are not in liquid form (e.g., ointment, gels) are also placed in a plastic container or on a nonadherent pad that is clearly labeled

Essential Facts

Preprinted labels for medications can help staff clearly label containers and syringes of medications. On the preprinted label it is optimal to include the concentration, if possible, when only one concentration is used. Otherwise, the concentration will have to be added manually to the preprinted label.

DISPOSING OF MEDICATIONS

At the end of the surgical procedure, any unused medications should be disposed of according to local, state, and federal regulations and the guidelines set forth by the individual organization.

Some common ways to dispose of medications include:

- Flushing down acceptable drains
- Empty vials sorted into specific disposal bins
- Incineration of specific medications
- Returning to pharmacy
- Returning to manufacturer

HANDLING OF CHEMOTHERAPY AGENTS

Chemotherapy agents are carcinogenic, mutagenic, or teratogenic antineoplastic agents and pose a health risk if the perioperative team is exposed to them.

Some common cytotoxic agents used include:

- Mitomycin
- Biodegradable polymers

- Methotrexate
- Cytarabine

Many of these drugs are administered in the operating room by way of:

- Bladder instillation (intravesical)
- Intracranial instillation
- Intrathecal (space around the spinal cord) instillation

The perioperative team must be aware of the hazards of chemotherapy and properly administer these medications safely. Common safety practices include:

- Medications are prepared in the pharmacy.
- Transportation of medication is done in a sealed and leak-proof container that is properly labeled.
- Personal protective equipment (PPE) is worn while handling medication, which includes a mask with a fluid shield, impervious or chemotherapy-rated gown, and two pairs of sterile gloves.
- Disposable instruments are used to administer chemotherapy in order to decrease exposure.
- Any unused chemotherapy or supplies used during the administration are discarded in the proper disposal container, which is commonly a biohazard container labeled "cytotoxic waste."

Essential Facts

Question: An intrathecal administration of methotrexate is required and you are the scrub nurse. What PPE should you be wearing?
Answer: You should wear a mask with a fluid shield, impervious or chemotherapy-rated gown, and two pairs of sterile gloves.

References

Institute for Safe Medication Practices. (2019). *Recommendations: List of confusing drug names*. Retrieved from https://www.ismp.org/recommedations/confused-drug-names-list

Tariq, R. A., Vashisht, R., & Scherbak, Y. (2021). Medication errors. StatPearls [Internet].

16

Anesthesia

Most surgical procedures in the operating room require some form of anesthesia. The perioperative nurse plays an important role in working collaboratively with the anesthesia provider and must be aware of the principles associated with anesthesia.

During this part of your orientation, you will learn about:

- The types of anesthesia
- The American Society of Anesthesiologists (ASA) classifications of physical status
- The levels of sedation/anesthesia and phases of anesthesia
- Monitoring of the patient
- The role of the circulating nurse
- Specific concerns during use of anesthesia

TYPES OF ANESTHESIA

The ASA considers anesthesia on a continuum of states of consciousness. There are four main types of anesthesia:

- General anesthesia
- Regional anesthesia
- Moderate/deep-sedation analgesia
- Local with/without monitored anesthesia care (MAC)

General Anesthesia

General anesthesia is a drug-induced state of unconsciousness, whereby there is no awareness or sensation. This type of anesthesia requires mask ventilation or intubation, as the patient may or may not be able to breathe on his or her own. The mode of administration is dependent on the level of anesthesia and the state of paralysis.

There are three phases of general anesthesia:

- Induction—when medications are given and the airway is secured
- Maintenance—when inhalation agents and/or medications are used to maintain an appropriate level of anesthesia
- Emergence—when the patient emerges from anesthesia at the end of the procedure

Medications Used for Induction

Medications will vary depending upon the preferences of the anesthesia provider, the type of anesthesia, the patient's physiologic status, and comorbidities.

Medications can be

- Inhalation gases
- Intravenous (IV)

Common inhalation gases used include:

- Air
- Oxygen
- Nitrous oxide
- Desflurane
- Sevoflurane

Common IV medications used include:

- Diazepam
- Midazolam
- Propofol
- Fentanyl

Common muscle relaxants used include:

- Succinylcholine (for rapid onset)
- Rocuronium (for rapid onset and intermediate duration)
- Cisatracurium (for intermediate onset)
- Vecuronium (for longer onset)

Neostigmine is a common reversal agent for a muscle relaxant that is combined with glycopyrolate to prevent bradycardia.

Airway Management Equipment

An airway can be safely managed with the following equipment:

- Nasal oxygen cannula
- Mask
- Endotracheal (ET) tube
- Laryngeal mask airway (LMA)

To secure an airway during general anesthesia, it is important to have several items available:

- Suction
- Oral airway
- Laryngoscope
- ET tube or LMA
- Stylet (can be placed in the lumen of the ET tube to make it more rigid)
- Tape
- GlideScope

A GlideScope is a video laryngoscope that provides visualization of the airway to assist in difficult intubations.

ET tubes can be:

- Cuffed
- Uncuffed (common in pediatrics)

ET tubes come in many sizes; choice of tube size depends on the size of the patient's trachea, ranging from 2.5 up to 8 mm.

Nasal Intubation

Sometimes, due to the type of surgery and the need to access the mouth, instead of orally intubating a patient, the patient may require the tube to be introduced into the nose and then extend down the nasopharynx into the trachea.

It is important to have several items available:

- Warm water to soften the ET tube
- Copious amount of lubricant
- McGill forceps (Figure 16.1) to navigate the tube into place
- Flexible scope for better visualization
- Nasal airway
- Vasoconstriction nose drops to limit bleeding and clear nasal passage

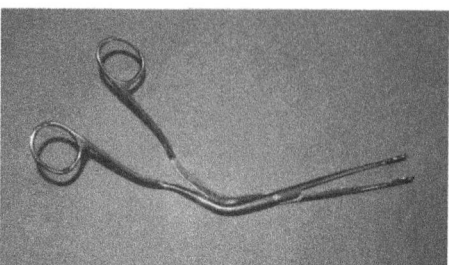

Figure 16.1 McGill forceps.

Essential Facts

Question: What are some of the items that should be available for intubation?
Answer: At minimum: a laryngoscope, suction, oral airway, ET tube or LMA, and tape should be available, as well as McGill forceps and lubricant if a nasal intubation.

Regional Anesthesia

Regional anesthesia is a loss of sensation to a specific part of the body, whereby local anesthesia medication is injected and blocks the nerves in that area. The blocks can be placed in different locations, for example:

- Spinal (subarachnoid space in spine)
- Epidural (epidural space in spine)
- Caudal (sacrum, for patients under 8 years old)
- Peripheral (extremities)

Many times, unless contraindicated, sedation accompanies the regional anesthesia to keep the patient comfortable and unable to hear what is going on in the environment (e.g., drilling during orthopedic surgery).

Common medications used for regional anesthesia are:

- Lidocaine
- Bupivacaine
- Fentanyl
- Morphine

Moderate-/Deep-Sedation Analgesia

Moderate-/deep-sedation analgesia occurs when the patient receives IV medication and is at a level of anesthesia whereby he or she can respond purposefully to verbal commands and will respond to light tactile stimulation. Usually, an airway or breathing assistance is not required.

Common medications used for moderate-/deep-sedation analgesia include:

- Diazepam
- Fentanyl
- Propofol

Local With/Without MAC

Local anesthesia is the infiltration, or topical application of medication, to a specific part of the body. When an anesthesia provider supplements local anesthesia with IV sedation while monitoring the patient's status, this is MAC, which is commonly used for minor procedures.

Common medications used for local anesthesia include:

- Lidocaine
- Bupivacaine

DETERMINING TYPE OF ANESTHESIA

To determine which type of anesthesia will be administered, the anesthesia provider must discuss the choices with the patient and surgeon. Factors that can influence this choice include:

- Type of surgery and duration of surgical procedure
- Surgeon preference
- Patient preference
- Patient's health status and history
- Positioning during surgery

ASA CLASSIFICATION OF PHYSICAL STATUS

The ASA uses a grading system to determine the physical status of a patient preoperatively to assess how the patient will tolerate the anesthesia. This status rates patients in six classes:

- ASA class 1—normal healthy patient
- ASA class 2—patient with mild systemic disease (e.g., well-controlled hypertensive, well-controlled diabetic, smoker)

- ASA class 3—patient with severe systemic disease (e.g., COPD, morbid obesity, pacemaker)
- ASA class 4—patient with severe systemic disease that is a constant threat to life (e.g., recent MI, CVA, TIA, cardiac stents)
- ASA class 5—moribund patient who is not expected to survive without the operation (e.g., ruptured abdominal/thoracic aneurysm, massive trauma, intracranial bleed)
- ASA class 6—declared-brain-dead patient whose organs are being removed for donor purposes

Essential Facts

Question: The patient being examined by the anesthesia provider prior to surgery states that he has mitral valve prolapse. Which ASA class would he be considered?
Answer: The patient would be considered ASA class 2, as mitral valve prolapse is a controlled disease of one body system.

MONITORING OF THE PATIENT

There are standard monitoring guidelines set forth by the ASA. The perioperative team should be aware of these guidelines and be able to apply them to monitoring the patient. Monitoring may include:

- Blood pressure
- Pulse oximetry
- ECG
- Heart rate
- Temperature
- Peripheral nerve stimulator (if muscle relaxants were used)
- Capnography (carbon dioxide concentration)
- Precordial or esophageal stethoscope (to assess breath sounds)
- Inspired oxygen analyzer
- Respirometer
- Low-pressure disconnection alarm

Suctioning

An assortment of suction catheters and tips should always be available for any type of anesthesia. It is common to start with Yankauer suction to eliminate oral secretions upon induction. Then a nasogastric tube may be used to suction any stomach content/secretions. This will prevent aspiration during emergence from anesthesia.

Essential Facts

The incidence of aspiration during anesthesia in adults is approximately three per 10,000 cases and in children is approximately four per 10,000 cases. Rates as high as 10 per 10,000 cases have been reported in children. It is important to always have suction available to the anesthesia provider at all times.

ROLE OF THE CIRCULATING NURSE DURING USE OF ANESTHESIA

The circulating nurse works closely with the anesthesia provider throughout the surgical procedure. Some common roles of the circulating nurse are:

- Assist with the placement of IV line and monitors.
- Stay at the right of the patient during induction to lend an extra hand (e.g., pass ET tube, pass suction, connect tube).
- Apply cricoid pressure, if necessary.
- Assist with blood administration.
- Remove monitors at the conclusion of surgery.
- Reorient patient after anesthesia.

Cricoid Pressure

At the beginning and end of a surgical procedure, the patient may be at risk of aspiration. Sometimes, due to the patient's physiological status (e.g., pregnancy) or dietary status (e.g., full stomach), a rapid-sequence induction is required. This involves the circulating nurse applying cricoid pressure while the anesthesia provider intubates the patient.

It is crucial that the nurse understands where and how to perform the Sellick maneuver (also known as *cricoid pressure*; Figure 16.2).

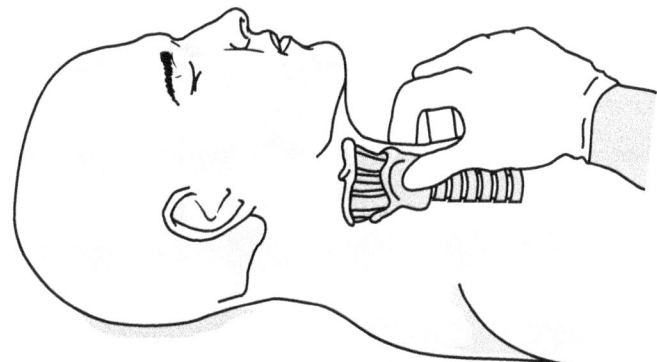

Figure 16.2 Cricoid pressure.

Procedure for applying cricoid pressure:

- Apply downward pressure on the cricoid cartilage with the thumb and index finger of the right hand (if standing on right of patient).
- Keep constant, firm pressure until the anesthesia provider states that pressure can be released, which will be after the ET tube is in place, cuff inflated, placement verified, and secured with tape.
- Releasing prematurely can cause the stomach contents to come up and go into the respiratory tract.

SPECIFIC CONCERNS DURING ANESTHESIA USE

Malignant Hyperthermia

Malignant hyperthermia (MH) is a specific concern commonly related directly to the administration of general anesthesia. MH is a potentially fatal inherited disorder that is linked to the administration of inhalation anesthetics and/or the muscle relaxant succinylcholine. This disorder is an acceleration of metabolism in skeletal muscles and exhibits the following initial signs and symptoms:

- Tachycardia
- Increased carbon dioxide level
- Muscle rigidity
- High body temperature (usually occurs later on)

An in-depth explanation of MH is provided in Chapter 17.

Essential Facts

The incidence of MH in children is one in 15,000 and in adults is one in 500,000. MH affects all ethnic groups, but males under 18 years of age have a higher incidence.

Pediatric Concerns

There are specific concerns relative to pediatric anesthesia. Some such concerns are:

- Monitors must be adapted to the size of the child for accuracy.
- Usually, children 8 years and under are induced with inhalation agents.
- Usually, patients over 8 years of age are induced with IV agents.

- A parent may accompany a child into the operating room to decrease anxiety.
- Normothermia must be maintained.

Geriatric Concerns

There are specific concerns relative to geriatric anesthesia administration. Such concerns are:

- Slower circulation of medications that can have a slower onset and may take longer to metabolize
- Loss of hearing that may cause difficulties with communication during emergence
- Maintenance of normothermia
- Skin integrity (e.g., use of gel headrest to prevent pressure sores)

17

Complications and Emergencies in the Operating Room

An emergency can present at any moment in the operating room setting. It is important to be armed with the knowledge and competency to quickly assess and provide treatment to the surgical patient. Some common emergencies in the operating room include motor vehicle accidents resulting in various injuries (e.g., ruptured spleen, cranial bleeding, or broken bones), ruptured aortic aneurysm, and intestinal obstruction.

During this part of your orientation, you will learn about:

- Assessment of the patient during an emergency
- Counting instruments and surgical supplies during an emergency
- Administration of blood products
- The crash/code cart
- Malignant hyperthermia (MH)
- Specialty situations

ASSESSMENT OF THE PATIENT

It is critical to assess the surgical patient in an emergent situation quickly to determine exactly what will be needed to render the appropriate treatment.

The basic assessment should include evaluation of:

- Airway
- Breathing
- Circulation
- Pain
- Neurological status
- Dietary status (NPO [nothing by mouth] status)

Vital signs and lab values should be monitored, and any critical or abnormal results should be reported immediately to the anesthesia provider and/or surgeon.

Surgical procedures that are most life-threatening should be performed first, and then the procedures should occur from cleanest (e.g., sterile) to dirtiest (e.g., contaminated).

Additional considerations in emergency situations include:

- Placement of urinary catheter to monitor urine output
- Availability of blood products
- Warming or cooling of patient
- Placement of arterial line or central line

COUNTING INSTRUMENTS AND SURGICAL SUPPLIES

If a patient is critically ill, the nurse should not take time away from the care of the patient to perform an instrument count. If possible, an attempt to count items (e.g., sponges, sutures, knife blades) should be taken. Also, only x-ray-detectable items should be used on the sterile field.

Regardless of what was counted or uncounted, once the patient is stabilized and surgery is concluded, a portable x-ray should be taken and read by a radiologist to ensure that there is no retained surgical item. Documentation should accurately reflect the emergency and inability to count surgical items.

ADMINISTRATION OF BLOOD PRODUCTS

Many different types of blood products may be administered in an emergency due to blood and fluid loss. Some common blood products include:

- Packed red blood cells (RBCs)
- Fresh frozen plasma
- Platelets
- Cryoprecipitate

The administration of blood products requires a crossmatching of a sample of the patient's blood to determine blood type and red cell antibodies.

Administration of blood products usually requires:

- A formal checking process prior to transfusion and a qualified second-person verification
- Use of correct equipment depending on the blood product (e.g., filter, tubing)
- Use of a blood warmer to keep the blood at body temperature
- Transfusion documentation

Complications of administration of blood products must be reported immediately and can include:

- Fever, chills, and urticaria (hives)
- Acute hemolytic transfusion reaction
- Contamination of blood products

Essential Facts

Question: To administer a unit of RBCs, what are some things you must gather?
Answer: You must gather the blood product, blood tubing, filter if needed, transfusion paperwork, blood warmer, and a qualified person to verify the administration process with you.

CRASH CART FOR SURGICAL EMERGENCIES

The crash cart, also known as *code cart*, is strategically located within the operating room semi-restricted area in case of an emergency. It is important to be familiar with the items found on the cart and how to use the defibrillator.

Common items in a crash cart include:

- Emergency medications
- Intravenous (IV) solutions
- 20- to 60-mL syringes
- Central venous catheter
- Arterial blood gas (ABG) collection device
- ECG electrodes
- Cut-down kits for arterial line
- Arterial line kit
- Suction catheters

Emergency Medications

Some common emergency medications for adults contained in the crash cart include:

- Amiodarone, 150-mg IV injection
- Atropine, 0.5- to 1-mg IV injection
- Calcium chloride, 0.5- to 1-mg IV injection
- Dopamine, 800-mg vial reconstituted in 500-mL IV bag of D5W (dextrose 5% in water) or normal saline
- Epinephrine, 1:10,000 1-mg IV injection
- Lidocaine, 100-mg/5-mL syringe for injection
- Lidocaine, 2-g vial reconstituted in 500-mL IV bag of D5W or normal saline
- Sodium bicarbonate, 50-mEq/50-mL syringe
- Epinephrine injection 1:1,000 0.3 mg
- Narcan 0.4-mg/1-mL to 0.8-mg IV injection

Some of these medications may come in prefilled syringes to make them easier and quicker to administer. *All dosages of medications should be checked and confirmed with the providers.*

Pediatric Considerations

Many times, because the dosage of medications and the size of supplies are so different for pediatric patients, a separate and distinct crash cart will be maintained for pediatric patients.

This crash cart can be:

- The same as for adults, but with age- and size-appropriate equipment, supplies, and medications
- A Braselow cart with resuscitation equipment, supplies, and medications

Essential Facts

A Braselow cart contains a special color-coded system that individualizes equipment and medication dosage relative to the patient's body length. This allows the perioperative team to concentrate on the emergency rather than on drug calculations and sizing an airway.

Defibrillator

The defibrillator is commonly housed on the top of the crash cart and can be used to electrically shock the heart of the surgical patient during cardiac arrest to help reestablish a normal rhythm.

A cardiac arrest includes heart rhythms such as:

- Asystole (Figure 17.1)
- Ventricular fibrillation (Figure 17.2)
- Pulseless ventricular tachycardia (Figure 17.3)
- Pulseless electrical activity

Resuscitating (defibrillation) a patient can be accomplished by:

- Applying defibrillator pads to the patient's chest (Figure 17.4)
- Placing external defibrillator paddles on the patient's chest
- Placing internal defibrillator paddles directly on the patient's heart

Table 17.1 describes defibrillator settings.

Cardiopulmonary resuscitation is continued throughout the emergency, if warranted, and medications are given until the patient is stabilized.

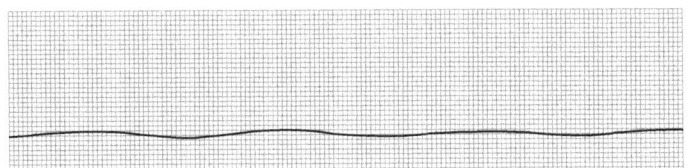

Figure 17.1 Asystole.

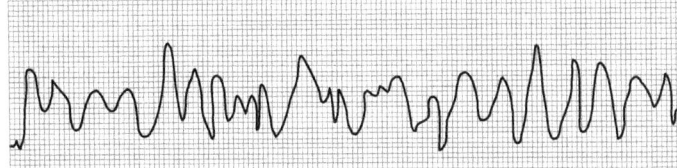

Figure 17.2 Ventricular fibrillation.

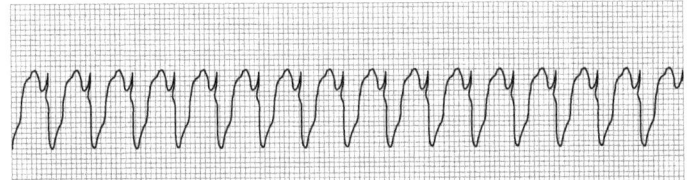

Figure 17.3 Pulseless ventricular tachycardia.

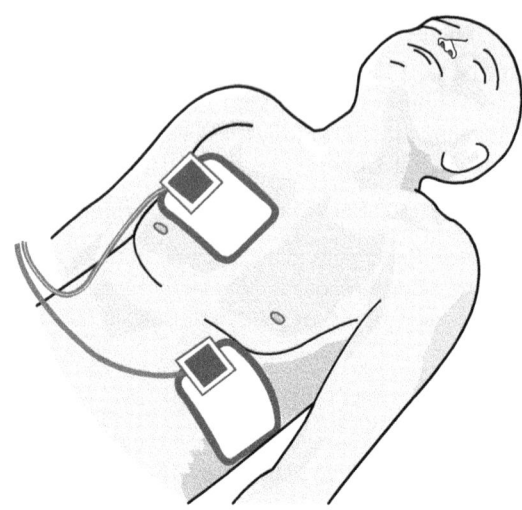

Figure 17.4 Placement of defibrillator pads.

Table 17.1

Defibrillator Settings

	External Pad/Paddle	Internal Paddle
Adult	120–200 J (biphasic) 200–360 (monophasic)	< 50 J
Child	2 J/kg of weight (biphasic and monophasic)	5–50 J

Essential Facts

The difference between a monophasic and biphasic defibrillator is in how the electrical energy passes through the patient. It is important to keep in mind that with a monophasic defibrillator, the settings are commonly higher.

Additional Testing

Additional laboratory and other types of testing equipment may be required to evaluate the status of the patient. Some common additional tests may include:

- ABGs (to check the acidity [pH] and the levels of oxygen and carbon dioxide in the blood)
- Pericardiocentesis (due to cardiac tamponade, when fluid builds up around the heart due to increased pressure)
- Electrolytes (to determine imbalance and subsequent treatment)
- Cardiac enzymes (to look at enzymes and proteins to determine how much damage has occurred to the heart)

MALIGNANT HYPERTHERMIA

MH is a specific concern commonly related directly to the administration of general anesthesia. MH is a potentially fatal, inherited disorder that is linked to the administration of inhalation anesthetics and/or the muscle relaxant succinylcholine. Therefore, it can manifest as a result of the patient receiving:

- Inhalation anesthesia (e.g., desflurane, enflurane)
- Succinylcholine

This is considered an emergency because, if left undetected and ultimately untreated, it can cause circulatory collapse, and possibly death, in a very short amount of time.

MH risk factors to consider are:

- It is unusual in the very young and very old.
- Males are affected more than females.
- Patients with trismus (lockjaw) have a higher incidence of positive MH testing.
- Of patients with trismus, 20% progress to MH after succinylcholine.
- Patients with some musculoskeletal disorders are at higher risk.

A thorough preoperative screening can help identify potential patients who may exhibit signs and symptoms of MH or be at risk of MH. Common questions to ask patients include:

- Is there a family history of MH?
- Have there been unexpected deaths or complications from anesthesia?
- Is there a personal history of high fever, muscle disorder, or dark-colored urine following anesthesia?

The classic presentation of MH in the operating room includes:

- Tachycardia (rapid heart rate)
- Rapid rise in end-tidal (ET) CO_2

- Cardiac arrhythmia
- Acidosis
- Hyperkalemia
- Rigidity

The early signs that should cause the certified surgical technologist (CST), RN, or first assistant concern are:

- Tachycardia and tachypnea (rapid breathing)
- Rapid rise in $ETCO_2$
- Sustained jaw rigidity
- Rapid exhaustion of soda lime that "turns blue"
- Hot soda lime canister

Soda lime is a mixture of chemicals that is used as a filter on the anesthesia machine. This filter removes the CO_2 from the breathing circuit. When the patient's CO_2 is elevated, the soda lime that is commonly white will turn blue, due to the rapid removal of CO_2. The soda lime canister will also feel hot to the touch.

The treatment for MH includes:

- Discontinue offending agents.
- Hyperventilate with 100% O_2.
- Give dantrolene sodium 2.5 mg/kg push, repeat as needed (PRN [pro re nata]).
- Treat hyperkalemia (bicarbonate 1–2 mEq/kg PRN).
- Cool the patient (gastric lavage, ice packs around patient or in wound).
- Measure arterial and/or venous blood gases.
- Obtain electrolytes and coagulation studies.

The Malignant Hyperthermia Association of the United States provides a hotline and detailed information on its website to assist healthcare providers in crisis with patients who have MH. It is important to have this information readily available in each operating room.

1-800-MH-HYPER
1-800-644-9737
www.mhaus.org

Essential Facts

Question: What is the treatment for an MH crisis?
Answer: Discontinue agent, hyperventilate with 100% O_2, give dantrolene sodium 2.5 mg/kg push IV, and cool the patient using ice packs and/or gastric lavage.

SPECIALTY SITUATIONS

Numerous specialty situations can present as an emergency in the operating room. Some such specialty situations are:

- Bullet removal
- Contraband removal
- Multiple-site injuries
- Medical anti-shock trouser (MAST) suit removal

Bullet Removal

- Bullets should not be handled with metal instruments or placed in metal containers due to the chance of scratching the bullet or compromising the surface.
- Once the bullet is removed and placed in a nonmetal container, it should be submitted to the police as per local and state law enforcement requirements.
- If there is an ongoing criminal investigation, the patient's clothing and belongings may also be secured as evidence. Therefore, the clothing should be cut off the patient prior to surgery along the seams and/or around the bullet- or stab-wound hole. These items should be placed in a paper bag to prevent moisture and growth of mold, which may potentially destroy or compromise the integrity of the evidence.
- Patient statements should also be documented accurately and in detail. Care should be taken to establish the chain of custody of the bullet and any other evidence from point of removal to examination by pathology and law enforcement.

Contraband Removal

Contraband is considered to be drugs, homemade weapons, and other illegal paraphernalia. These items can come into the operating room hidden in patient body cavities. It is important to:

- Place the contraband in a plastic container, so as to not compromise its integrity.
- Submit contraband to the police as per local and state law enforcement requirements.
- Secure the patient's clothing and belongings as evidence in the event of a criminal investigation.
- Document accurately the patient's statements in detail and establish the chain of custody of the contraband and any other evidence from point of removal to examination by pathology and law enforcement.

Multiple-Site Injuries

Multiple-site injuries may require multiple teams of surgeons working on the patient simultaneously. Therefore, these procedures may require multiple scrub RNs/CSTs and multiple circulating nurses. It is important to delegate tasks appropriately to maximize assistance. Also, priority will be given to the most life-threatening injuries. This decision will be made by the anesthesia provider and surgeon.

MAST Garment Removal

An MAST (medical anti-shock trouser) garment, also known as military anti-shock trouser or pneumatic anti-shock garment, may be used on patients for trauma situations such as hypovolemic shock. This compression garment is placed from the patient's rib line to the ankles and should be inflated if the patient is hypotensive. When removing the MAST garment prior to emergency surgery, it is important to remember that it should not be cut off the patient, but rather deflated while monitoring the blood pressure to prevent a sudden drop in blood pressure or shock.

End-of-Life Care

At the end of life, care should be taken to consider the cultural and religious beliefs of the individual patient.

Some considerations are:

- Call clergy.
- Have an organ donation representative available to discuss donor opportunities.
- Provide appropriate comfort measures for the patient.
- Provide a designated area for the family to gather privately with the patient.
- Have a palliative care provider available to answer questions.

Essential Facts

There are three circumstances in which organs can become available for procurement: patient death determined by neurological criteria (brain death), by circulatory or cardiopulmonary criteria, or by voluntary donation, such as a healthy patient donating a kidney. It is becoming more common to allow family in the OR after circulatory

(continued)

(*continued*)

or cardiopulmonary criteria have been met and the patient is being removed from life support and waiting to die, prior to the procurement of the organs. Because OR staff are commonly advocating for patients and performing life-saving measures, family presence may create anxiety and an uncomfortable feeling for the staff. However, it can help families begin the healing process by knowing that they have created a positive outcome through organ donation (Gysin, Khairallah, & Reef, 2015).

Reference

Gysin, D. M., Khairallah, T. S., & Reef, M. (2015). Donation after circulatory death: Simulating and implementing family presence in the OR. *OR Nurse*, *9*, 29–36.

18

Emergency Preparedness for Disaster

"In failing to prepare, you are preparing to fail." Benjamin Franklin

During this part of your orientation, you will learn about:

- Collaboration efforts before, during, and after a disaster
- Types of disasters
- Ways to prepare for a disaster

A disaster can occur at any time and it is imperative to have a planned response. This response should be on a personal, family, community, and organizational level. All hospitals should have an Emergency Operations Plan (EOP). This plan describes how a facility will respond to and recover from any type of emergency. It is important that the hospital collaborate with the community to prepare for a disaster. During any disaster, the hospital will set up an Incident Command Center or an Emergency Operations Center. This center will manage, control, and synchronize the emergency response within the hospital and with responding agencies. Any emergency requires a collaborative effort.

LEVELS OF COLLABORATION AND COMMUNICATION

The public deserves collaborative leadership before, during, and after a catastrophic event maintaining a standard of responsiveness with effective coordination of resources. There are a multitude of public, nonprofit, and private entities intimately involved in a disaster that require communication and coordination.

Some entities involved in a disaster:

- Hospital
- Fire department
- Police department
- Local governmental agencies (municipalities, school districts)
- Federal agencies (FEMA)

Levels of communication:

- Horizontal (transmission of communication at the same level)
- Vertical (transmission of communication to different levels in a hierarchy)

Communication within any organization should cascade down from senior leadership to all areas of the organization. This communication should be specific and have structure so that personnel receive timely notifications. Announcements can be made via many different types of systems:

- Public address system (overhead intercom)
- Pager system
- Emergency telephones (Cellular, satellite telephone, or emergency radio)
- Face-to-face

Communication style should be:

- Clear with a consistent message
- Precise and timely
- Ongoing during and after the disaster

SETTING UP A TEAM

Any level of communication requires teams to be established that should be multi-disciplinary in effort to represent all key stakeholders. Within the perioperative setting and hospital, some of the key stakeholders should include personnel from:

- Anesthesia department
- Material management
- Safety and security
- Central sterile processing

- Surgical booking office
- Nursing
- Ancillary services
- Pharmacy
- Environmental services
- Infection prevention
- Risk management
- Engineering department
- Wellness services to support staff

Roles in the operating room during a disaster should be assigned to individuals that possess the position and skill set to successfully navigate the disaster. Most often, elective surgery is placed on hold or delayed, and the staff will be reassigned. The staff will assume the role that is assigned to them by the perioperative leader (Table 18.1).

ID badges must be worn by all personnel, so that they are identifiable, as well as employees should be checked in to work daily to maintain accurate records when needing to locate a person during an emergency. Also, current contact information, as well as emergency contact information, should be up to date within the hospital human resource system.

Table 18.1

Roles During a Disaster	
Perioperative leader	Usually a nurse manager or their designee who will be communicating with the command center and coordinating any and all surgical responses.
Scribe	An individual that will keep notes on all communication with names and times of all events.
Specialty coordinator	A staff nurse or surgical technologist that helps to coordinate specific supplies, physicians, and staff that will be operating.
Staff coordinator	A staff nurse or designee that will assign and track staff assignments, as well as identifying when additional staff will be needed, break time will be authorized, or when staff is overstressed.
Anesthesia lead	Usually an anesthesia provider that will help triage patients and coordinate the anesthesia team.
Surgeon lead	Usually the chief of surgery that works with the team to coordinate the surgeons, triage patients, and communicate to the medical staff.

> **Essential Facts**
>
> Some ID badges are now being made with Smart Chips or RFID Technology so responders can react efficiently during an emergency and identify who is missing and where they are. This can provide a faster response time and ultimately save lives.

TYPES OF DISASTERS

Emergency situations are a constant threat facing the United States healthcare system, as well as communities around the world. There are specific responses for different types of disasters, especially those that involve a large number of people (mass casualty).

Types of disasters:

- Natural disaster (i.e., flood, hurricane, tornado)
- Man-made disaster (i.e., riot, chemical attack, biological attack, bombing)

> **Essential Facts**
>
> Natural disasters alone kill on average 60,000 people per year, globally.
> Question: What can you do to prepare for a disaster?
> Answer: Create a personal plan, know your hospital EOP, participate in a drill.

Location of disaster:

- Internal- in the facility such as a power outage or fire
- External- outside the facility such as multi-injury car accident or terror attack

Some man-made disasters require facility-based decontamination of staff or patients that are exposed to chemical, biological, or radiological materials (Table 18.2). There are three areas for decontamination to focus upon:

- Decontamination and treatment of a specific agent
- Determination when decontamination is sufficiently completed
- Prehospital decontamination

The Occupational Safety and Health Administration (OSHA) regulates and requires protection of workers based upon the specific

Table 18.2

Factors Affecting Decontamination

Contact time	Amount of time the material is in contact
Concentration	The level of concentration and permeation of material
Temperature	The higher the temperature usually increase permeation of material
Physical state	Gases, vapors, and low-viscosity liquids usually permeate quicker

exposure material. Facilities maintain safety data sheets that identify each chemical, as well as the physical, health, and environmental health hazards, the protective measures, and the required safety precautions for handling, storing, and transporting the chemical. This should be consulted when an exposure occurs.

Some chemical agents include:

- Nerve agents (i.e., Sarin, Tabun, Soman)
- Blood agents (i.e., Hydrogen cyanide, Cyanogen chloride)
- Heavy metals (i.e., Arsenic, Lead, Mercury)

Some biological contaminants include:

- Anthrax
- Plague
- Botulism

Some radiological materials include:

- Radiological dispersal device (RDD) or "dirty bomb"
- Nuclear-generator release or detonation
- Medical radiation misuse or failure

Mass casualty

Mass casualty events have grown around the world especially since the New York City terror attacks on September 11, 2001. These events require healthcare works to mobilize quickly, making the best decision for the individual event and circumstance. The operating room is relied upon heavily to respond quickly and appropriately.

Types of mass casualties include:

- Terrorist attacks
- Mass shootings
- Violent crimes

BECOMING PREPARED

The Joint Commission has required organizations to take on an "all hazards" approach to disaster planning by reviewing and analyzing all credible threats to a community. This requires all healthcare facilities to participate in, at minimum, one emergency drill a year that includes all four phases of disaster management (Table 18.3).

Strategies for success:

- Create clear guidance for personnel
- Clearly define roles and schedules
- Establish a framework for communication
- Plan to brief and update team members on status
- Communicate with other areas of the hospital (PACU)
- Learn from past events and drills

Performance metrics help drive success, improve quality, and assure patient safety. Many metrics are measured during normal circumstances with defined performance targets, but it is important to compare these metrics to disaster circumstances in effort to benchmark against other institutions during similar events. Some meaningful indicators for comprehensive assessment of hospital emergency management include:

- Surgical patient volume
- Emergency Department length of stay
- Wait times for patients
- Equipment functionality

Table 18.3

Phases of Disaster Management:		
Phase	Description	Example
Mitigation	identify potential emergency and implement a plan	creation of a policy and procedure
Preparedness	develop activities to learn how to manage an emergency	written plan for staffing, supplies, and triage of patients
Response	develop activities to control the negative effects from an emergency	participate in a drill, tabletop discussion, review of plan
Recovery	restore essential services and resume normal operations	reschedule surgeries, replenish supplies

- Overall patient volume
- Hospital wide length of stay
- Morbidity and mortality rates

Resources

There are many excellent resources available to help you with emergency preparedness. Some resources are:

- http://www.fema.gov/media-library/assets/documents/89550
- https://www.ready.gov/business/implementation
- https://training.fema.gov/is/
- https://www.jointcommission.org/resources/patient-safety-topics/emergency-management/
- https://www.cdc.gov/phlp/publications/topic/hospital.html
- https://www.osha.gov/SLTC/emergencypreparedness/index.html
- https://cdp.dhs.gov/find-training/course/PER-902
- https://www.euro.who.int/__data/assets/pdf_file/0008/268766/Hospital-emergency-response-checklist-Eng.pdf
- https://healthcareready.org/cms-emergency-preparedness-knowledge-center/

References

AORN. (2020). *Emergency and disaster preparedness tool kit.* https://aorn.org/guidelines/clinical-resources/tool-kits/emergency-preparedness-tool-kit

ARB. (2020). *RFID emergency management and evacuation tracking.* https://www.abr.com/rfid-emergency-management-evacuation-tracking/

CovidSurg Collaborative. (2020). Global guidance for surgical care during the COVID-19 pandemic. *Journal of British Surgery, 107 no.9 (2020): 1097-1103*

Davis, S. S. (2018). The key to safety: Preparing for disasters. *AORN Journal, 108*(3), 233–235.

Koenig, K. L., Boatright, C. J., Hancock, J. A., Denny, F. J., Teeter, D. S., Kahn, C. A., & Schultz, C. H. (2008). Health care facility-based decontamination of victims exposed to chemical, biological, and radiological materials. *The American Journal of Emergency Medicine, 26*(1), 71–80.

Our World in Data. (2019). *Natural disasters.* https://ourworldindata.org/natural-disasters

Spruce, L. (2019). Back to basics: Mass casualty incidents. *AORN Journal, 109*(1), 95–103.

The Joint Commission. (2020). *Emergency management standard.* https://www.jointcommission.org/standards/prepublication-standards/emergency-management-standard-em030103-revisions/

19

Legal Aspects of Operating Room Practice

Malpractice litigation has risen substantially in the past few decades. There are there are approximately 200,000 preventable hospital-related deaths each year in the United States (Kavanagh, Saman, Bartel, & Westerman, 2017). Medical malpractice cases account for approximately $10 billion in costs to healthcare providers each year. A great deal of time, expense, and energy is spent on malpractice claims and litigation. Patient safety and nursing vigilance play a key role in decreasing error and decreasing the chance of litigation.

During this part of your orientation, you will learn about:

- Common operating room complications that lead to litigation
- Ways to limit malpractice exposure
- The anatomy of a lawsuit
- Common legal terms and principles

COMMON OPERATING ROOM COMPLICATIONS THAT LEAD TO LITIGATION

Common complications that lead to litigation in the operating room are:

- Medication error
- Retained surgical item (RSI)

- Wrong-site surgery
- Surgical burn (e.g., electrocautery burn)
- Positioning complications

WAYS TO LIMIT MALPRACTICE EXPOSURE

There are some important ways to limit malpractice exposure. These include:

- Accurate, timely, and complete nursing documentation
- Incident reporting
- Abiding by policies and procedures of the organization
- Staying focused on the job and minimizing distractions

Nursing Documentation

Anything that is transcribed on paper, printed, or electronically generated into the patient's record must be accurate, timely, and complete. Accurate documentation is the best way to defend against a legal claim related to nursing care.

Documentation must be:

- Factual
- Objective
- Complete
- Relevant
- Confidential
- Concise

Patient care information must be secure, confidential, and protected from unauthorized disclosure. Therefore, it is imperative not to share patient information and potentially breach the Health Insurance Portability and Accountability Act (HIPAA), which mandates the privacy of patients receiving healthcare and the confidentiality of their health information.

Incident Reporting

An *incident* is an event that occurs that is not routine or normal. The incident reporting system informs the risk management department of the event, so that the hospital can assess the situation from a legal standpoint and provide additional support. This may require the organization to publicly report the incident or possibly institute a corrective measure to prevent future incidents. Various states may require incident reporting as part of their public health statutes.

Incidents can be:

- Actual
- Near miss
- Potential injury
- Good catch

Some incidents may require or result in a health department investigation or other municipal/governmental investigation. Therefore, it is imperative to accurately report the incident in a timely fashion.

Essential Facts

Question: The surgery is over and the RN notices a reddened area under the electrosurgery unit (ESU) ground pad site. Should the RN complete an incident report?

Answer: Because this is not a normal occurrence, the RN should complete an incident report to notify the risk management department of the event. It should also be reported to the surgeon and the nurse manager. Documentation should be completed on the chart, and follow-up and documentation should occur in the post-anesthesia care unit. The redness may simply be a reaction to the grounding pad, but it must be documented and observed. The redness may also be a surgical burn.

Policies and Procedures

Policies and procedures are unique to each organization and are based on evidence in the literature. Policies and procedures should be routinely reviewed by an interprofessional team. Most often, intraoperative policies are created by using the Association of peri-Operative Registered Nurses's *Guidelines for Perioperative Practice* (2021) and other recommendations set forth by other regulatory agencies (e.g., Occupational Safety and Health Administration, Centers for Disease Control and Prevention).

ANATOMY OF A LAWSUIT

A lawsuit has many parts, and the language associated with each part can become confusing. The person/party who initiates the lawsuit is the *plaintiff*. The person/party being sued is the *defendant*.

The basic anatomy of a lawsuit has four common phases:

- Pleadings phase—This refers to the formal allegation by the plaintiff to the institution and/or doctor that begins the

actual lawsuit, consisting of a complaint and followed by an answer.
- Discovery phase—this is the interrogation back and forth between the plaintiff and the defendant (e.g., institution and/or doctor) and production of records and documents, commonly consisting of depositions.
- Pretrial phase—if a settlement is not reached, preparation to go to trial begins.
- Trial phase—Most cases settle or may be discontinued before this point, but if an agreement cannot be reached between the plaintiff and the defendant, a jury may be chosen and a trial will begin, and the verdict will bring closure to the case.

Prerequisites for a Medical Malpractice Claim

There are two prerequisites to a medical malpractice claim that are necessary to prevail in a lawsuit:

- The plaintiff/patient must establish through expert testimony a departure from acceptable medical standards and practice occurred.
- The plaintiff/patient must prove that the departure constituting the medical malpractice is the proximate cause of the injury and/or death.

Statutes of Limitations

The time in which a plaintiff/patient can commence an action for medical malpractice is governed by the individual laws of each state. Considerations that affect the statute of limitations include:

- Age and competency of the plaintiff (e.g., infant or competency of the plaintiff)
- The nature of the claim or malpractice (e.g., negligent acts, RSI, intentional acts)
- The precise title, licensing professional, or type of specialty (e.g., licensed physician, technician, nurse)
- The corporate status or structure of the institution (e.g., municipal hospital, private hospital)

Because statutes of limitations are the result of each state's legislation, every state can potentially have different time periods for legal action. Furthermore, under federal law in matters governed by Medicare/Medicaid regulations or malpractice actions against federal medical facilities, there may be additional time periods to consider.

COMMON LEGAL TERMS AND PRINCIPLES

Common legal terms and principles in medical malpractice lawsuits include:

- *Res ipsa loquitor*
- *Respondeat superior*
- Lack of informed consent

Res Ipsa Loquitor

The theory of *res ipsa loquitor*, Latin for "it speaks for itself," eliminates the two elements listed earlier that are required to be proven in a lawsuit. In circumstances in which the medical provider has exclusive control, and there is no other possible explanation, the plaintiff can prove the case without the departure prerequisite.

Examples of *res ipsa loquitor* are:

- Retention of a surgical item (e.g., sponge, instrument)
- Burns received during surgery

Respondeat Superior

For RNs, certified surgical technologists, and RN first assistants working within the employment of a hospital, the doctrine of *respondeat superior* is applicable. This concept provides protection to medical provider employees in the event they are involved in a lawsuit within the scope of their employment. This does not apply to independent contractors (e.g., private physicians).

Employees will be provided defense costs (e.g., legal representation) and indemnification (e.g., insurance coverage) for the lawsuit.

The bases of the claim must arise from one of the following:

- Conduct
- Acts
- Omissions

Actions outside the scope of employment (e.g., assault, fraud) would be excluded from *respondeat superior*.

Essential Facts

Question: A hospital nurse is off duty and renders nursing care to a pedestrian at the site of a motor vehicle accident. Is the nurse covered under the doctrine of respondeat superior?

Answer: No, the nurse is not covered because he was not working within the employment of the hospital.

Lack of Informed Consent

Various state statutes govern the requirements for informed consent before any procedure is performed on a patient. In addition to the medical malpractice actions, there is commonly a claim for lack of informed consent.

Informed consent commonly requires that the patient understands:

- The procedure itself
- The risks of the procedure
- The benefits of the procedure
- The alternatives to the procedure

The informed consent must be provided in layperson's terms and be in a language that the patient understands. If it is not, a translating device (e.g., phone interpretation device) must be used.

Before the patient signs the consent, the patient must be afforded:

- Time to review the consent
- Time to ask questions

Essential Facts

If a patient undergoes a surgical procedure without a signed consent, in some states this can be construed as an assault under the state's penal codes.

References

Association of periOperative Registered Nurses. (2021). *Guidelines for perioperative practice*. Denver, CO: Author.

Kavanagh, K. T., Saman, D. M., Bartel, R., & Westerman, K. (2017). Estimating hospital-related deaths due to medical error: A perspective from patient advocates. *Journal of Patient Safety, 13*(1), 1–5.

20

Lifelong Learning

"Intellectual growth should commence at birth and cease only at death."—Albert Einstein

During this part of your orientation, you will learn about:

- Ways lifelong learning can be accomplished
- Resources to access for learning
- The need for creating mentoring experiences

No truer words were spoken by Albert Einstein since operating room nurses are always learning and the operating room is a practice setting that will always provide an opportunity to learn. The American Association of Colleges of Nursing and the Association of American Medical Colleges described a vision for the future of continuing education and lifelong learning for healthcare professionals that emphasizes interprofessional, team-based, innovative, learner-centered teaching methods with collaboration from academia, healthcare, accrediting bodies, licensing and credentialing boards, as well as others associated within the healthcare systems (Kroning, 2016).

Lifelong learning can be accomplished through many different venues that vary with time and commitment. Some such venues for learning include:

- Learning resources and tools
- Credentialing
- Higher education

Since an effective surgical team depends on the knowledge, skills, and qualifications of its members, it is vital that learning is an ongoing process. There are many different resources and tools that can be utilized to sustain your personal professional goals and to provide optimum, evidence-based care to the patient.

LEARNING RESOURCES AND TOOLS

Types of learning resources and tools:

- In-service training
- Conferences and seminars
- Online education

In-service training

Most organizations provide weekly or monthly in-service training to update staff regarding the latest developments in practice, process, or new equipment. This training is commonly conducted by a nurse educator, nurse manager, or a representative from the company that provide the equipment.

In-services can provide the following types of learning:

- Didactic information
  - Annual updates
  - Clinical information
  - Process or policy information
- Active learning
  - Return demonstration is observed by the leader to learn a new skill
- Simulation
  - Provides a realistic, context-rich experiential learning in a safe environment
  - Uses standardized patients
  - Can utilize low and high fidelity mannequins or a virtual world

Conferences and seminars

Conferences and seminars are excellent opportunities to exchange ideas and insights with leaders in a particular field and then to return to your organization with the tools and resources to implement change. This forum for learning can contain similar types of learning to in-service training, but the networking that occurs is invaluable. The networking can be in-person or virtual, which can be more efficient and global.

Types of conferences and seminars

- Institutional sponsored
- Local chapter meetings
- Regional conferences
- National conferences
- International conferences/seminars

Conferences and seminars are opportunities for networking. Networking at all levels provides an opportunity for nurses and CSTs to discuss current issues with subject experts, speakers, and vendors, while forging new relationships with staff members from other organizations. Most often, you will return to your practice with inspiration and new enthusiasm. Also, it is important that information that is gleaned from the conference and seminar is brought back to your practice setting and shared with your colleagues that did not attend. The dissemination of new knowledge creates rich and evidence-based practice settings, especially in the operating room.

Online Education

Online education is a popular mode of learning since the learner can accomplish this in a synchronous or asynchronous environment. This makes it easier to schedule around work, family, and personal obligations. There are many online education opportunities that are free or sometimes have a fee, which are most often needed to maintain your license or certification.

Online education can be in the form of:

- Continuing education online and live courses
- Continuing education journal articles
- Online or live webinars
- Toolkits that address critical patient safety issues

Essential Facts

Read your current journals. To date, there are approximately 262 nursing journals in circulation (Nurse Author and Editor, 2019). Some nursing journals are broad, and some are within a given specialty. It is important to note within the operating room what journals are most read, consulted, and cited. This will give you an idea of what journal you should subscribe to on an annual basis. Journal subscription provides a great way to stay up to date on what is happening currently in the operating room. AORN Journal is one such journal that is the go-to for perioperative resources.

There are specific educational programs (Periop 101) provided through AORN that are designed to recruit, educate, and retain perioperative nurses that are new graduates, nurses transitioning into the perioperative suite from other nursing specialties, and other surgical team members. There are also more advance courses (Periop 202) that concentrate on specialty surgical procedures. These types of programs are based in evidence and provide theory that is essential for safe patient care. Many organizations utilize these specialized resources to have the most up to date information and guidelines for practice.

CREDENTIALING

Credentialing is another way to be a lifelong learner and continue your education. There are many different perioperative nursing credentials.

Some of the perioperative nursing credentials include

- CNOR (Certified Nursing in the Operating Room)
- CRNFA (Certified Registered Nurse First Assist)
- CSSM (Certified Surgical Services Manager)
- CNS-CP (Clinical Nurse Specialist- Certified Perioperative) for masters-prepared Clinical Nurse Specialists
- CNAMB (Certified Ambulatory Surgery Nurse) (AORN, 2020)

Nurses that pursue a certification through a specific agency that validates the nurse's knowledge, skills, and abilities in a specific role and clinical area of practice tend to have a feeling of personal accomplishment, institutional recognition, and have career advancement opportunities. Most often associated with maintaining a certification, a stipend of money is provided that can assist in defraying the cost of continuing education expenses. It also shows a commitment to exceptional patient safety and adherence to current standards.

Most often certifications are renewed every 5 years by either recertification examination or the completion of a specific amount of continuing education that is specific to the practice setting. This demonstrates the continuing dedication to excellence, current commitment to specialized knowledge, and a personal obligation to patient safety.

Essential Facts

Specialty nurse certification is clearly linked to the improved quality of patient care and more positive patient outcomes. Certification

(continued)

(continued)

also enhances nurse confidence, empowerment, and increased job satisfaction (Whitehead et al., 2019). There are more than 40,000 nurses internationally that proudly hold the CNOR credential, which is a personal and professional accomplishment (CCI, 2020).

Higher Education

Higher education is another path that can be taken by the operating room nurse to gain new knowledge or to help secure a higher position in an organization. There are many different career paths that can lead to administrative, educational, or leadership positions. All of these positions commonly require a higher degree than a Bachelor of Science in Nursing.

Higher education degrees include:

- Masters of Science in Nursing (MSN)
- Masters in Business Administration (MBA)
- Doctorate of Education (EdD)
- Doctorate of Philosophy (PhD)
- Doctorate of Nursing Practice (DNP) (AACN, 2020)

The choice of degree is a personal choice that should be based upon review of the curricula, coupled with projected career path and personal desire, as well as where you see yourself in 5 years, 10 years, and 20 years. There needs to be deep reflection and an honest assessment of your goals, while making a realistic choice dependent upon your responsibilities, since the delivery of higher education can range from onsite, virtual or even hybrid. Base the choice of delivery method upon how you learn best. Do you prefer a synchronous environment that you attend at a specific date and time, or do you prefer learning asynchronously where you can carve out bits of time in your day to learn? Everyone is different and should assess their personal strengths, as well as look at their own personal responsibilities.

Some resources of interest below can help you along your educational journey to lifelong learning. There is no cookie-cutter path for anyone, which makes it more of an adventure. As a lifelong learner, you can always reinvent yourself over time and move in a different direction when you feel that you are looking to develop in a different direction. The perioperative area has many opportunities that can fit different lifestyles and diverse goals. It is all up to your preference and perseverance towards your goals.

Some resources Conferences and seminars

- https://www.aorn.org/search#q=conference
- https://www.ormanager.com/events/
- https://surgical.nursingconference.com/events-list/perioperative-surgical-nursing

Online education and Continuing Education

- https://www.aorn.org/aorn-journal/aorn-journal-ce-articles
- https://www.pfiedlereducation.com/diweb/start
- https://www.nurse.com/ce/perioperative-nursing
- https://www.aorn.org/education/facility-solutions/periop-101/or
- https://www.aorn.org/education/facility-solutions/periop-202

Credentialing

- https://www.aorn.org/education/individuals/credentialing
- https://www.cc-institute.org/
- https://nascertification.com/crnfa/
- https://www.cc-institute.org/cssm/learn/
- https://www.cc-institute.org/cns-cp/learn/
- https://www.cc-institute.org/cnamb/learn/

Higher Education

- https://www.aacnnursing.org/Nursing-Education-Programs/Masters-Education
- https://www.aacnnursing.org/Nursing-Education-Programs/DNP-Education
- https://www.aacnnursing.org/Nursing-Education-Programs/PhD-Education

MENTORSHIP

Mentorship is an important consideration that can promote professional development and lifelong learning. Mentoring can be

- informal (i.e., non-established relationship that can be short-term or long-term)
- formal (i.e., structured relationship with specific objectives)

Mentoring should not be confused with having a preceptor. A preceptor is a predetermined person that is teaching a skill or a task. A preceptor is important in the operating room to learn new procedures or new techniques, and is short term. A mentor is someone who is knowledgeable and established in the field with the goal of developing the mentee on a personal and professional level.

Operating room nurses at all levels can find mentors that can help them to develop professionally. These mentors may not be within their organization or within nursing. Sometimes it is beneficial to find a mentor in another discipline. Do not be afraid to ask someone to be a mentor. Most often, mentorship is advantageous to both the mentor and the mentee.

Steps to finding a mentor:

1. Observe staff members or leaders that have qualities you would like to gain information, advice, and knowledge from.
2. Go outside of nursing and determine if any other people could be potential mentors.
3. Determine your short-term and long-term goals of this mentorship relationship.
4. Discuss the potential mentorship relationship with the chosen person.
5. Establish a mentoring schedule that is conducive for both parties.
6. Celebrate small accomplishments.

Essential Facts

Question: What is your elevator pitch?

When looking for a mentor, you need to have your elevator pitch. This is a short informative statement that conveys your professional ambitions, highlights your objectives, and explains why this mentorship relationship would be beneficial. This statement should be practiced and exude firmness and confidence, while being constructive.

Benefits to mentorship:

- Provides guidance and support
- Helps build confidence
- Cultivates clinical decision-making
- Fosters empowerment
- Supports career development and networking

A mentorship is a special relationship that should be nurtured and valued. Over time, when one mentor relationship ends, another one may begin, as well as you may become the mentor and be able to give back to your profession in an invaluable way.

References

AORN. (2020). *Education*. https://www.aorn.org/education/individuals/credentialing

AACN. (2020). *Nursing education programs*. https://www.aacnnursing.org/Nursing-Education-Programs

CCI. (2020). *Learn about certifications*. https://www.cc-institute.org/

Kroning, M. (2016). Lifelong learning in nursing. *Journal of Christian Nursing, 33*(1), 60. https://doi.org/10.1097/CNJ.0000000000000235

Nurse Author and Editor. (2019). Directory of nursing journals. https://nursingeditors.com/journals-directory/

Whitehead, L., Ghosh, M., Walker, D. K., Bloxsome, D., Vafeas, C., & Wilkinson, A. (2019). The relationship between specialty nurse certification and patient, nurse and organizational outcomes: A systematic review. *International Journal of Nursing Studies, 93*, 1–11.

Bibliography

American Association of Tissue Banks. (2017). *Standards for tissue banking* (14th ed.). McLean, VA: Author.

American Heart Association. (2020). *Advanced cardiovascular life support provider manual* (16th ed.). South Deerfield, MA: Channing L. Bete.

American Institute of Architects. (2018). *Guidelines for design and construction of hospital and health care facilities.* Dallas, TX: Facility Guidelines Institute.

American Society of Anesthesiologists, House of Delegates. (1999, October 13). Continuum of depth of sedation—Definition of general anesthesia and levels of sedation/analgesia (last amended October 15, 2014). Retrieved from http://www.asahq.org

American Society of Anesthesiologists Task Force on Prevention of Perioperative Peripheral Neuropathies. (2011). Practice advisory for the prevention of perioperative peripheral neuropathies: An updated report. *Anesthesiology, 114*(4), 741–754.

American Society of Anesthesiologists Task Force on Sedation and Analgesia by Non-Anesthesiologists. (2002). Practice guidelines for sedation and analgesia by non-anesthesiologists. *Anesthesiology, 96*(4), 1004–1117.

American Society of Health-System Pharmacists. (2015). ASHP guidelines on outsourcing sterile compounding services. *American Journal of Health-System Pharmacy, 72*, 1664–1675.

Anderson, D. J. (2014). Prevention of surgical site infection: Beyond SCIP. *AORN Journal, 99*(2), 315–319.

Standard, A.N.S.I., and A.A.M.I. ST79. "Comprehensive guide to steam sterilization and sterility assurance in health care facilities." *Association for the Advancement of Medical Instrumentation/American National Standards Institute* (2017).

Association for the Advancement of Medical Instrumentation. (2015). *Sterilization, Part 1: Sterilization in health care facilities Volume 1.* Annapolis Junction, MD: Advancing Safety in Medical Technology Publications.

Association of Operating Room Nurses. (2021). *Guidelines for Perioperative Practice 2021*. Denver: CO: AORN

Association of periOperative Registered Nurses. (2021). AORN comprehensive surgical checklist. Retrieved from http://www.aorn.org/guidelines/clinical-resources/tool-kits/correct-site-surgery-tool-kit/aorn-comprehensive-surgical-checklist

Association of periOperative Registered Nurses. (n.d.). AORN safe patient handling pocket reference guide. Retrieved from https://www.aorn.org/-/media/aorn/guidelines/tool-kits/safe-patient-handling/safe-patient-handling-pocket-reference-guide.pdf?la=en&hash=54A3288EDE43FF121FF94AC4257960CAD67B68C5

Association of Surgical Technologists. (2010). AST standards of practice for ionizing radiation exposure in the perioperative setting. Retrieved from http://www.ast.org/uploadedFiles/Main_Site/Content/About_Us/Standard%20Ionizing%20Radiation%20Exposure.pdf

Barash, P. G., Cullen, B. F., & Stoelting, R. K. (2015). *Clinical anesthesia* (7th ed.). Philadelphia, PA: Lippincott Williams & Wilkins.

Bashaw, M. A. (2016). Guideline implementation: Processing flexible endoscopes. *AORN Journal, 104*(3), 225–236.

Bhatt, A., Mittal, S., & Gopinath, K. S. (2016). Safety considerations for Health care Workers involved in Cytoreductive Surgery and Perioperative chemotherapy. *Indian Journal of Surgical Oncology, 7*(2), 249–257.

Bouyer-Ferullo, S. (2013). Preventing perioperative peripheral nerve injuries. *AORN Journal, 97*(1), 110–124.e9. doi:10.1016/j.aorn.2012.10.013

Burcharth, J., & Rosenberg, J. (2013). Animal derived products may conflict with religious patients' beliefs. *BMC Medical Ethics, 14*(1), 48.

Centers for Disease Control and Prevention. (2016). Guidance for the selection and use of personal protective equipment (PPE) in healthcare setting. Retrieved from http://www.cdc.gov/HAI/prevent/ppe.html

Centers for Disease Control and Prevention. (2017). Guidelines for preventing surgical site infections. Retrieved from https://www.cdc.gov/infectioncontrol/guidelines/ssi/index.html

Cherry, B., & Jacob, S. R. (2016). *Contemporary nursing: Issues, trends, & management* (7th ed.). St. Louis, MO: Elsevier Health Sciences.

Covidien. (2013). Principles of electrosurgery. Retrieved from http://www.asit.org/assets/documents/Prinicpals_in_electrosurgery.pdf

Criscitelli, T. (2016). Caring for patients with chronic wounds: Safety considerations during the surgical experience. Association of operating room nurses. *AORN Journal, 104*(1), 67.

Davis, P. J., & Cladis, F. P. (2016). *Smith's anesthesia for infants and children* (9th ed.). New York, NY: Elsevier.

Falk, S. A., & Fleisher, L. A. (2020). Overview of anesthesia. In S. B. Jones (Ed.) *UpToDate*. Retrieved from https://www.uptodate.com/contents/overview-of-anesthesia

Fencl, J. L. (2017). Guideline implementation: Surgical smoke safety. *AORN Journal, 105*(5), 488–497.

Food and Drug Administration. (2014). Medical device tracking—Guidance for industry and Food and Drug Administration staff. Retrieved from https://www.fda.gov/downloads/MedicalDevices/DeviceRegulation andGuidance/GuidanceDocuments/UCM071775.pdf

Hicks, R. W. (2014). Understanding medication compounding issues. *AORN Journal*, *99*(4), 466–479.

Hopper, W., & Moss, R. (2010). Common breaks in sterile technique: Clinical perspectives and perioperative implications. *AORN Journal*, *91*(3), 350–367.

Institute for Safe Medication Practices. (2021). ISMP list of high-alert medications in acute care settings. Retrieved from http://www.ismp.org/Tools/institutionalhighAlert.asp

James, J. T. (2013). A new, evidence-based estimate of patient harms associated with hospital care. *Journal of Patient Safety*, *9*(3), 122–128.

Kenters, N., Huijskens, E. G., Meier, C., & Voss, A. (2015). Infectious diseases linked to cross-contamination of flexible endoscopes. *Endoscopy International Open*, *3*(04), E259–E265.

Kohn, L. T., Corrigan, J. M., & Donaldson, M. S. (Eds.). (2000). *To err is human: Building a safer health system*. Washington, DC: National Academies Press.

Liang, P., Yu, J., Lu, M.-D., Dong, B.-W., Yu, X.-L., Zhou, X.-D., . . . Lu, G.-R. (2013). Practice guidelines for ultrasound-guided percutaneous microwave ablation for hepatic malignancy. *World Journal of Gastroenterology*, *19*(33), 5430–5438.

Malignant Hyperthermia Association of the United States. (2021). What is malignant hyperthermia? Retrieved from http://www.mhaus.org

Nanji, K. C., Patel, A., Shaikh, S., Seger, D. L., & Bates, D. W. (2016). Evaluation of perioperative medication errors and adverse drug events. *Journal of the American Society of Anesthesiologists*, *124*(1), 25–34.

Occupational Safety and Health Administration. (2011). OSHA fact sheet: Personal protective equipment (PPE) reduces exposure to blood borne pathogens. Retrieved from http://www.osha.gov/OshDoc/data_BloodborneFacts/bbfact03.pdf

O'Grady, N. P., Alexander, M., Burns, L. A., Dellinger, E. P., Garland, J., Heard, S. O., . . . Weinstein, R. A. (2011). *Guidelines for the prevention of intravascular catheter-related infections*. Atlanta, GA: Centers for Disease Control and Prevention.

Phillips, N. & Hornacky, A. (2020). *Berry & Kohn's operating room technique* (14th ed.). St. Louis, MO: Elsevier Health Sciences.

Putnam, K. (2015). Guideline for prevention of retained surgical items. *AORN Journal*, *102*(6), P11–P13.

Ray, M. J., Lin, M. Y., Weinstein, R. A., & Trick, W. E. (2016). Spread of carbapenem-resistant Enterobacteriaceae among Illinois healthcare facilities: The role of patient sharing. *Clinical Infectious Diseases*, *63*(7), 889–893.

Rothrock, J. C. (2018). *Alexander's care of the patient in surgery* (16th ed.). St. Louis, MO: Elsevier.

Spruce, L. (2017). Back to basics: Sterile technique. *AORN Journal*, *105*(5), 478–487.

Squeo, R. (2015, July 21). WISCA. Top clinical concerns related to surgical gloves. Retrieved from http://www.wisc-asc.org/news/242516/Top-Clinical-Concerns-Related-to-Surgical-Gloves.htm

Zimlichman, E., Henderson, D., Tamir, O., Franz, C., Song, P., Yamin, C. K., ... Bates, D. W. (2013). Health care-associated infections: A meta-analysis of costs and financial impact on the US health care system. *JAMA Internal Medicine*, *173*(22), 2039–2046.

Index

abdominal aortic aneurysm resection, 100
abdominal procedures, 100–102
    drapes for, 100
    positions for, 100
    supplies for, 100
absorbent natural sutures, 85
absorbent synthetic sutures, 86
adjunct count technology, 119
adrenergic agonists, 150
adults
    emergency medications for, in crash cart, 168
    lab tests for, 17–18
advanced bipolar energy, 133–134
    blades/tips, 134
    characteristics of, 133
    components of, 133
    generator settings, 133
    safety considerations, 134
    surgical procedures using, 134
airborne precautions, 56–57
airway management equipment, 157
alcohol, 36–37, 52
American Association of Tissue Banks, 91
American National Standards Institute, 106
American Pharmacists Association, 149
American Society of Anesthesiologists (ASA)
    classification of physical status, 159–160
    monitoring of patient, guidelines, 160–161
amiodarone, 168
anesthesia, 155–163
    American Society of Anesthesiologists classification of physical status, 159–160
    circulating nurse during use, role of, 161–162
    cricoid pressure, 161–162
    determine type of, 159
    general, 156–158
    local with/without monitored anesthesia care, 159
    moderate/deep-sedation analgesia, 158–159
    monitoring of patient, 160–161
    suctioning, 160
    provider, role of, 60
    regional, 158
    specific concerns during, 162–163
        geriatric concerns, 163
        malignant hyperthermia, 162
        pediatric concerns, 162–163
    types of, 155–159

ankle stirrups, 29–30
anthrax, 181
antibiotics, for preoperative conditions, 14
appendectomy, 100
argon, 106
argon-enhanced electrosurgery, 125
arthroscopy, 103
Association of periOperative Registered Nurses, 106, 129, 149
atropine, 168

Bacillus stearothermophilus, 77
Bacillus subtilis var. niger, 77
balanced salt irrigating solution (BSS), 97–98
beach chair. *See* semi-Fowler's position
biodegradable polymers, 152
biological contaminants, 181
biphasic defibrillator, 170
bipolar circuit, 124–125
bladder tumor, 102
bleeding
    hemoclips for, 138
    herbal supplements increasing, 16
blepharoplasty, 97
blood products, administration of, 166–167
body sheet, 96–97
boot stirrups, 29–30
botulism, 181
Bowie-Dick tests, 77
Braselow cart, 168
bronchoscopy, 98
BSS. *See* balanced salt irrigating solution
bullet removal, 173
bupivacaine, 158–159

calcium chloride, 168
Carbon dioxide, 106
carbon dioxide gas, 101
cardboard bridge, 97

cardiac, thoracic, and vascular procedures, 98–100
    drapes for, 98
    positions for, 98
    specialty equipment, 99
    supplies for, 99
cardiac arrest, 168–170
cardiopulmonary resuscitation, 169–170
casting, 144–145
    application of, 144
    material, 144
    splints, 145
cataract surgery, 97
catheters, 88–89
cavitation, 132
cefazolin, 14
Centers for Medicare and Medicaid Services, 13
certified surgical technologist (CST), 42, 52, 60, 150, 172, 189
    preparing operating room for surgery, 60
    role in transferring medications, 151
chemotherapy agents, handling of, 152–153
chest drainage system, 99
chest tube, 99
CHG. *See* chlorhexidine gluconate
CHG with alcohol, 36–37
chlorhexidine gluconate (CHG), 13, 36
cholecystectomy, 100
circulating nurse, role of
    in preparing operating room, 60
    in transferring medications, 151
    during use of anesthesia, 161–162
cisatracurium, 156
clamping/grasping instruments, 111–113
    clamps, 112
    forceps, 112–113
    needle holders, 113
closed-glove technique, 66–67
Clostridium difficile, 56–57
colon resection, 100

confusing names, of medications, 150
consent form, 18
contact precautions, 55–56
contraband removal, 173
coronary artery bypass graft, 98
counting instruments, requirements for, 117–119
    adjunct count technology, 119
    methods for, 118
    resolving count discrepancies, 118
    risk of retained surgical items, 118
cranioplasty, 104
craniotomy, 104
crash cart, 167–171
    medications for adults in, 168
    for pediatric patients, 168
    for surgical emergencies, 167–171
cricoid pressure, 161–162
cryoablation, 135–136
    components of, 135
    safety considerations, 136
    surgical procedures using, 136
    use, 136
cryotherapy machine (retinal procedures), 98
CST. *See* certified surgical technologist
cuff hands, 43–44
cutting/dissecting instruments, 110–111
cytarabine, 153
cytotoxic agents, 152–153

dacrocystorhinostomy, 97
decontamination, 180–181
    chemical agents, 181
    factors affecting, 181
decontamination, equipment for, 72
defendant, 187–188
defibrillator, 168–170
    placement of pads, 170
    settings, 169–170
detergent, 51–52

diazepam, 15, 156, 159
dilatation and curettage, 102
dilating/probing instruments, 114–116
disaster, emergency preparedness for, 177–183
    becoming prepared, 182–183
    collaboration and communication, levels of, 177–178
    entities involved in, 178
    location of, 180
    management, phases of, 182
    mass casualty in, 181
    roles during, 179
    team, setting up, 178–180
    types of, 180–181
discovery lawsuit phase, 188
disinfectants, 52
disposable eye knives and needles, 97
dopamine, 150, 168
Doppler ultrasound, 100
double gloving, 67
drains, 89
drapes, 41–47
    basic principles of, 43–44
    common order of, 44
    components of, 41–43
        fenestrated drape, 42
        plastic drape, 42
        sheet, 42
        stockinette, 42–43
        towels, 42
    goals of, 41
    infection control consideration, 45
    lead aprons, 46
    materials, choice of, 43
    other items in operating room, 46
    radiation badge, 47
    removal of, 45
    securing items to, 44–45
droplet precautions, 56
drug compounding, 149–150
dynamic air-removal steam sterilization, 79, 81

electrosurgery unit (ESU), 121–129
  components of, 121
  different tissue effects, 125–126
  hand-piece tips, 127
  methods of, 122–125
    argon-enhanced electrosurgery, 125
    bipolar circuit, 124–125
    foot pedal, 124–125
    ground pad (return electrode), 122–124
    monopolar, 122–124
    ultrasonic radiofrequency, 125
    vessel-sealing instruments, 125
  power settings on, 126
  safety considerations, 127–128
    alternate site burns, 128
    capacitive coupling, 128
    direct coupling, 128
    do nots of, 128
  settings, 126–127
  surgical smoke, evacuation of, 129
  tips, cleaning, 127
Emergency Operations Plan (EOP), 177
end-of-life care, 174
endotracheal tube (ET), 157
enucleation, 97
envelope-style wrapper, 61–63
Environmental Protection Agency (EPA), 51
environment requirements, of operating room, 51–58
  alcohol, 52
  assessing, 52–54
  cleaning, 51–52
    disinfectants for, 52
    products, 51–52
  humidity and air exchange, 54
  infection control precautions, 57
    airborne precautions, 56–57
    cleaning after, 57
    contact precautions, 55–56
    droplet precautions, 56
    standard precautions, 55
  noise in, 57–58
  temperature and airflow, 54
  traffic patterns, 54–55
  waste disposal, 58
enzymatic solution, 72–73
EOP. *See* Emergency Operations Plan
EPA. *See* Environmental Protection Agency
epinephrine, 150, 168
eschar, 127
ESU. *See* electrosurgery unit
ET. *See* endotracheal tube
ethylene oxide chemical
  advantages of, 81
  disadvantages of, 81
  parameters for, 79
  sterilization, 78
ET tubes, 157
excision of chalazion, 97
exenteration, 97
external fixator, 103

facial reconstruction, 95
femoral-popliteal bypass, 98
fenestrated drape, 42
fentanyl, 150, 156, 158–159
flammable preparation agents, 39
flexible endoscopes, handling of, 80
foot pedal, 124–125
forceps, 112–113
free tie, 86

general age-appropriate considerations, 104–105
general anesthesia, 156–168
  airway management equipment, 157
  medications used for
    induction, 156
    inhalation gases, 156
    intravenous medications, 156
    muscle relaxants, 156
  nasal intubation, 157–158
  phases of, 156
geriatric anesthesia, 163
GlideScope, 157

gloves, 64–65, 69–70
gown, 65–66, 69–70
gravity displacement steam sterilization, 78
ground pad (return electrode), 122–124
growth factors, 144
gynecological and genitourinary procedures, 102–103
   drapes for, 102
   positions for, 102
   supplies for, 102–103

hair removal, prior to skin preparation, 35–36
hand-rub technique, 64–65
Hank/Hegar dilators, 114–115
head coverings, 7–8
   bouffant style, 6
   do nots of, 6
   skull-cap style, 7
head drape, 96–97
healthcare-accredited laundering requirements, 5
Health Insurance Portability and Accountability Act (HIPAA), 186
hemoclips, 138
herbal supplements, 16
herniorraphy, 100
high-alert medications
HIPAA. *See* Health Insurance Portability and Accountability Act
hip replacement, 103
hydrogen peroxide plasma sterilization
   advantages of, 81
   disadvantages of, 81
   parameters of, 79
hydroxyzine, 15
hypothermia, 20
hysterectomy, 102

identification badges, 9
IED. *See* implanted electronic device

immediate-use steam sterilization (IUSS), 80–81
impedance, 122
implanted electronic device (IED), 124
implants, 90–91, 97
incident reporting
indicators, in sterilization process, 77
infection control concerns, 11
infection control precautions, 55–57
   airborne precautions, 56–57
   cleaning after, 57
   contact precautions, 55–56
   droplet precautions, 56
   standard precautions, 55
informed consent, 18–19
informed consent, lack of, 190
Institute for Safe Medication Practices (ISMP), 150
instruments. *See* surgical instrumentation
insufflation, 101
insulation failure, 128
iodine-based with alcohol, 36–37
ISMP. *See* Institute for Safe Medication Practices
IUSS. *See* immediate-use steam sterilization

jackknife (Kraske) position, 26–27
jewelry, 9
Joint Commission Board of Commissioners, 19

keratoplasty, 97
knee-crutch stirrups, 29–30
knee replacement, 103
knife blades, 84–85

lab work, 17–18
   factors, 17
   tests for adults, 17–18
laminectomy, 103
laparoscopic instruments, 116

laparoscopic procedures, 100–102
laparotomy (or lap) drape. *See* fenestrated drape
laser procedures, 98, 105–107
    guidelines for safety, 106–107
    interactions with tissue, 106
    laser energy, 106
    risk, 106
    types of laser, 106
laser safety officer, 106
lateral position, 29–31
    common position for, 31
    nerve injury in, 31
    positioning devices for, 31
    and skin breakdown in, 31
lawsuit, anatomy of, 187–188
lead aprons, 46
levofloxacin, 14
lidocaine, 158–159, 168
lithotomy position, 27–29
    common position for, 28
    levels of, 29
    nerve injury in, 28
    positioning devices for, 28–29
    and skin breakdown, 28
    stirrups, 29
litigation, complications leading to, 185–186
local anesthesia, 159
location of disaster, 180

MAC. *See* monitored anesthesia care
Malignant Hyperthermia Association of the United States
malignant hyperthermia (MH), 162, 171–172
    early signs, 162
    preoperative screening, 171–172
    presentation of, 172
    risk factors, 171
    treatment for, 172
malpractice exposure, ways to limit, 186–187
man-made disaster, 180
manual cleaning, 73
manufacturer's wrapper, 61–63
mass casualty in disaster, 181
mastectomy, 100
Mayo scissors, 111
McGill forceps
MDROs. *See* multiple-drug-resistant organisms
mechanical cleaning, 74
medical antishock trouser (MAST) garment removal, 174
medical malpractice claim, prerequisites to, 188
medications, 149–153
    chemotherapy agents, handling of, 152–153
    confusing names of, 150
    disposing of, 152
    handling and administration of, on sterile field, 151–152
    preparing, 149–150
    preprinted labels for, 152
    transferring of, 150–151
methicillin-resistant *Staphylococcus aureus* (MRSA), 56
methotrexate, 153
MH. *See* malignant hyperthermia
microscope drape, 97
microwave ablation, 136
    components of, 136
    generator settings, 136
    safety considerations, 136
    surgical procedures using, 136
midazolam, 15, 150, 156
mitomycin, 152
mitral valve replacement, 98
moderate-/deep-sedation analgesia, 158–159
moderate sedation agents
monitored anesthesia care (MAC), 155
monofilament suture, 86
monophasic defibrillator
monopolar methods, 122–124
morphine, 158
MRSA. *See* methicillin-resistant *Staphylococcus aureus*
multifeed stapling devices, 138
multifilament suture, 86

multiple-drug-resistant organisms (MDROs), 56
multiple-site injuries, 174
muscle relaxants, 156

narcan, 168
nasal intubation, 157
nasal reconstruction, 95
natural disaster, 180
natural sutures
　absorbent, 85
　nonabsorbent, 86
Nd:YAG, 106
neck dissection, 95
needle
　holders, 113
　sutures with, 85–87
　syringes and, 87–88
neuromuscular blocking agents
neurosurgery procedures, 104
　drapes for, 104
　positions for, 104
　supplies for, 104
noise, in operating room, 57–58
nonabsorbent natural sutures, 86
nonabsorbent synthetic sutures, 86
normothermic temperature, 20
nursing assessment, components of, 15–16

Occupational Safety and Health Administration (OSHA), 106, 180–181
open reduction internal fixation, 103
operating room (OR)
　complications/emergencies in, 165–175
　　additional testing, 170–171
　　assessment of patient, 165–166
　　blood products, administration of, 166–167
　　counting instruments and surgical supplies, 166
　　crash cart for surgical emergencies, 167–171
　　defibrillator, 168–170
　　emergency medications, 168
　　end-of-life care, 174
　　malignant hyperthermia, 171–172
　　pediatric considerations, 168
　　specialty situations, 173–175
　draping other items in, 46
　environment requirements, 51–58
　legal aspects of, 185–190
　medications, 168
　preparing, for surgery, 60
operating room practice, legal aspects of, 185–190
　complications leading to litigation, 185–186
　lawsuit, anatomy of, 187–188
　　limitations, statutes of, 188
　　medical malpractice claim, prerequisites to, 188
　　phases of, 187–188
　legal terms and principles, 189–190
　　informed consent, lack of, 190
　　res ipsa loquitor, 189
　　respondeat superior, 189
　ways to limit malpractice exposure, 186–187
　　incident reporting, 186–187
　　nursing documentation, 186
　　policies and procedures, 187
ophthalmic procedures, 97–98
　drapes for, 97
　positions for, 97
　specialty equipment, 98
　supplies for, 97
OR. *See* operating room
orthopedic procedures, 103–104
　drapes for, 103
　positions for, 103
　supplies for, 104
OSHA. *See* Occupational Safety and Health Administration

otolaryngology, head, and neck procedures, 95–97
  drapes for, 96
  positions for, 96
  supplies for, 96–97

parathyroidectomy, 95
patient positioning, 23–34
  additional considerations for safety, 33
  common positioning injuries, 24
  effective, goals of, 23
  ergonomic and safety for surgical team, 33–34
  factors put patients at risk for injury due to, 23–24
  general considerations for safe, 23–24
  protecting patient from pressure injuries, 24
  safety guidelines for, 24
  standard surgical positions, 25–33
    lateral, 29–31
    lithotomy, 27–29
    prone, 26–27
    supine (dorsal recumbent), 25–26
    Trendelenburg position, 31–33
pediatric anesthesia, 162–163
peel-and-seal package, 61–63
peracetic acid sterilization, 79
  advantages of, 81
  disadvantages of, 82
  parameters for, 79
peripherally inserted central catheter, 41
personal items, 10
personal protective equipment (PPE), 55–56, 72
phacoemulsification machine (cataract procedures), 98
physical status, grading system to determine, 159–160
plague, 181
plaintiff, 187–188
plastic drape, 42
pleadings lawsuit phase, 187–188
pneumonectomy, 98
pneumoperitoneum, 101
positioning injuries, 24
posterior vitrectomy machine (vitrectomy procedures), 98
povidone-iodine, 36–37
power of attorney, 18–19
PPE. *See* personal protective equipment
prednisone, 150
preoperative conditions, 13–21
  informed consent, 18–19
  lab work, 17–18
  medications for, 14–15
    antibiotics, 14
    sedatives, 14–15
  patient identifiers, 15
  preoperative questions, 15–16
  preoperative shower, 13–14
  preoperative teaching, 16–17
  preoperative warming, 20–21
  universal protocol, 19–20
    preprocedural verification, 19
    sign out, 20
    site marking, 19
    time out, 19–20
preoperative teaching, 16–17
pressure injuries, considerations for protecting from, 24
pretrial lawsuit phase, 188
prewarming, of patients, 20
probes, 115–116
prone position, 26–27
  common position for, 26
  nerve injury in, 27
  positioning devices for, 27
  safety considerations for, 27
  and skin breakdown, 27
propofol, 156, 159
prostatectomy, 102

radiation badge, 47
radiofrequency (RF) surgical energy, 134–135
  components of, 134

hand pieces, 135
low-temperature, 135
safety considerations, 135
surgical procedures using, 135
regional anesthesia, 158
reloads, 137-138
REM. *See* return electrode monitoring
res ipsa loquitor, 189
respondeat superior, 189
retained surgical items (RSIs), risk of, 117-119
retracting instruments, 113-114
return electrode, 122-124
return electrode monitoring (REM), 123
RF. *See* radiofrequency
rigid sterilization container, 63-64
robotic surgery, 103
rocuronium, 156
RSIs. *See* retained surgical items

saline, 151
salpingo-oophorectomy, 102
scissors, 110-111
scrub(s), 4-6
brush technique, 65
description of, 4
do nots of, 5
jackets, 7
laundering of, 5
nurse, role of, 60
soap choices, 64-65
sedatives, for preoperative conditions, 14-15
Sellick maneuver, 161-162; *See also* cricoid pressure
semi-Fowler's position, 96
sharps, 84-90
catheters, 88-89
drains, 89
knife blades, 84-85
other accessories, 90
sterile covers, 88
suction tubing, 88
sutures and needles, 85-87
syringes and needles, 87-88

sheet, draping, 42
shock position. *See* Trendelenburg position
shoe covers, 8
shoes, 8
silver-impregnated dressings, 143
skin antiseptic agent, 36-37; *See also* skin inspection
application of, 37
choosing correct, 36
locations of use and, 37
types of, 36-37
skin inspection, 36
skin preparation, 35-40
basic principles for, 37
general guidelines for, 38
goals of, 35
hair removal prior to, 35-36
hazards of, 38-39
skin antiseptic agent, 36-38
application of, 37-38
locations of use, 37
selection of, 36
types of, 36-37
skin inspection, 36
skin substitutes, 143-144
soda lime
sodium bicarbonate, 168
sodium chloride for injection, 150
soft silicone-bordered dressings, 143
specialty instruments, 117
spinal fusion, 104
splints, 145
split-thickness skin graft
sponges, 83-84
SSIs. *See* surgical site infections
standard precautions, 55
stapedectomy (middle ear procedure), 96
staplers, 137
choice of, 137
hemoclips, 138
reloads, 137-138
types of, 137
stapling devices, 137-138
hemoclips, 138
multifeed, 138

stapling devices (*cont.*)
  reloads, 137–138
  safety considerations for
  types of, 137–138
statutes of limitations, 188
steam sterilization, 78–82
  advantages of, 81
  disadvantages of, 81–82
  dynamic air removal, 79
  gravity-displacement, 79
sterile covers, types of, 88
sterile field, 63
  breaking down, 69–70
  setting up and maintaining, 68
  techniques for delivering items, 63
  transferring items to, during surgery, 68–69
sterile storage, 82
sterile technique, 59–70; *See also* sterilization
  closed glove technique, 66–67
  definition, 59
  determining sterility of items, 61
  general principles of, 59–60
  gowning, 65–66
  instrument packaging, types of, 63
  preparing operating room for surgery, 60
  removal of gown and gloves, 69–70
  scrubbing, 63–65
  sterile field, 68–70
    breaking down, 69–70
    setting up and maintaining, 68
    techniques for delivering items, 63
    transferring items to, during surgery, 68–69
  sterile supplies packaging, 61–63
sterile water, 151
sterilization, 77–82
  biological indicators for, 77
  chemical indicators for, 77
  cleaning and decontamination, 72–74
  enzymatic solution, 72–73
  final rinse of all instruments, 73–74
  instruments and equipment for, 72
  manual cleaning, 73
  mechanical cleaning, 74
  personal protective equipment for, 72
  ultrasonic cleaning, 73
  washer-decontamination cycles, 74
  flexible endoscopes, handling of, 80
  immediate-use steam sterilization, 80–81
  mechanical indicators for, 77
  preparation and packaging, 75–77
    indicators, 77
    items for inspection, 75
    packaging instruments, 76
    packaging materials, 76
    packaging requirements, 75–76
    specialty equipment, 76
  process flow, 71
  sterile storage, 82
  types of, 77–78
    advantages and disadvantages of, 81–82
    dynamic air-removal, 79
    ethylene oxide chemical, 79
    gravity-displacement steam, 78
    hydrogen peroxide plasma, 79
    immediate-use steam sterilization, 80–81
    peracetic acid, 79
stethoscopes, 9
stirrups, 29–30
stockinette, 42–43
succinylcholine, 150, 156
suction catheters, 160
suction tubing, 88
supine position, 25–26, 96
  common position for, 25
  nerve injury in, 26
  positioning devices for, 26
  and skin breakdown, 25–26

surgical attire, 3–11
　additional items, 9–11
　　identification badges, 9
　　jewelry, 9
　　masks, 10–11
　　personal items, 10
　　stethoscopes, 9
　controlled areas, 3–4
　　monitored unrestricted
　　　area, 4
　　restricted area, 3–4
　　semirestricted area, 4
　　transition area, 4
　head coverings, 6–7
　　bouffant style, 6
　　do nots of, 6
　　skull-cap style, 7
　infection control concerns, 11
　scrub jackets, 7
　scrubs, 4–6
　　description of, 4
　　do nots of, 5
　　laundering of, 5
　shoe covers, 8
　shoes, 8
surgical dressings, 139–145
　casting, 144–145
　　application of, 144
　　material, 144
　　splints, 145
　different types of, 141
　products for wounds, 142–144
　　growth factors, 144
　　silver-impregnated dressings, 143
　　skin substitutes, 143–144
　　soft silicone-bordered dressings, 143
　　wound VACs, 142–143
　purpose of, 140–141
　securing, 142
　surgical wound classifications, 139–140
　wound closure, types of, 140
surgical energy, 131–136
　advanced bipolar, 133–134
　cryoablation, 135–136
　microwave ablation, 136
　radiofrequency, 134–135
　types of, 131
　ultrasonic, 132–133
surgical instrumentation, 109–119
　clamping or grasping instruments, 111–113
　counting instruments, requirements for, 117–119
　cutting or dissecting instruments, 110–111
　dilating/probing instruments, 114–116
　instrument categories, 109–110
　laparoscopic instruments, 116
　retracting instruments, 113–114
　specialty instruments, 117
surgical inventory systems, 91–92
surgical masks, 10–11
surgical procedures, basics of, 95–107
　cardiac, thoracic, and vascular procedures, 98–100
　general age-appropriate consideration, 104–105
　general and abdominal procedures, 100–102
　gynecological and genitourinary procedures, 102–103
　head drape, 96
　laparoscopic procedures, 100–102
　laser procedures, 105–107
　neurosurgery procedures, 104
　ophthalmic procedures, 97–98
　orthopedic procedures, 103–104
　otolaryngology, head, and neck procedures, 95–97
　robotic surgery, 103
surgical site infections (SSIs), 13
surgical smoke, evacuation of, 129
surgical supplies, 83–92
　general guidelines for, 90
　implants, 90–91
　sharps, 84–90
　　catheters, 88–89
　　drains, 89
　　knife blades, 84–85
　　other accessories, 90

sterile covers, 88
suction tubing, 88
sutures and needles, 85–87
syringes and needles, 87–88
sponges, 83–84
surgical inventory systems for, 91–92
types of, 83–90
surgical team, ergonomic and safety considerations for, 33–34
sutures
characteristics, 85–87
natural
absorbent, 85
nonabsorbent, 86
with needles, 85–87
reel, 87
synthetic
absorbent, 86
nonabsorbent, 86
syringes, needles and, 87–88

TASS. *See* toxic anterior segment syndrome
terminal cleaning, 53
thermoluminescent dosimeter, 47
thoracotomy, 98
thyroidectomy, 95
thyroid gland, 46
tissue banks, 91
tissue effects, different, 125–126
tonsillectomy, 95
towels, 42
toxic anterior segment syndrome (TASS), 76
tracheal dilators, 114
traffic patterns, operating room, 54–55
transurethral resection of prostate
transurethral resection of prostate/badder tumor, 102
Trendelenburg position, 31–33
common position for, 32
nerve injury in, 32
positioning devices for, 32–33
and skin breakdown, 32
trial lawsuit phase, 188
trocars, 101–102
type 5 integrators, 77

U drape, 96–97
ultrasonic cleaning, 73
ultrasonic radiofrequency, 125
ultrasonic surgical energy, 132–133
blades/tips, 132–133
components of, 132
factors affecting, 132
generator settings, 132
safety considerations, 132
surgical procedures using, 133
universal protocol, 19–20
preprocedural verification, 19
sign out, 20
site marking, 19
time out, 19–20
urethral dilators, 114

vancomycin, 14
vancomycin-resistant enterococci (VRE), 56
vascular dilators, 114
vecuronium, 156
vessel-sealing instruments, 125
Vi-drape. *See* plastic drape
VRE. *See* vancomycin-resistant enterococci

washer-decontamination cycles, 74
waste disposal, 58
Weck-Cel, 97
wound classifications, 139–140
wound closure, types of, 140
wound VACs, 142–143

www.ingramcontent.com/pod-product-compliance
Ingram Content Group UK Ltd.
Pitfield, Milton Keynes, MK11 3LW, UK
UKHW021258180426
11947UKWH00015B/902